Addiction: A Very Short Introduction

VERY SHORT INTRODUCTIONS are for anyone wanting a stimulating and accessible way into a new subject. They are written by experts, and have been translated into more than 45 different languages.

The series began in 1995, and now covers a wide variety of topics in every discipline. The VSI library currently contains over 700 volumes—a Very Short Introduction to everything from Psychology and Philosophy of Science to American History and Relativity—and continues to grow in every subject area.

Very Short Introductions available now:

ABOLITIONISM Richard S. Newman
THE ABRAHAMIC RELIGIONS
   Charles L. Cohen
ACCOUNTING Christopher Nobes
ADDICTION Keith Humphreys
ADOLESCENCE Peter K. Smith
THEODOR W. ADORNO
   Andrew Bowie
ADVERTISING Winston Fletcher
AERIAL WARFARE Frank Ledwidge
AESTHETICS Bence Nanay
AFRICAN AMERICAN RELIGION
   Eddie S. Glaude Jr
AFRICAN HISTORY John Parker and
   Richard Rathbone
AFRICAN POLITICS Ian Taylor
AFRICAN RELIGIONS
   Jacob K. Olupona
AGEING Nancy A. Pachana
AGNOSTICISM Robin Le Poidevin
AGRICULTURE Paul Brassley and
   Richard Soffe
ALEXANDER THE GREAT
   Hugh Bowden
ALGEBRA Peter M. Higgins
AMERICAN BUSINESS HISTORY
   Walter A. Friedman
AMERICAN CULTURAL HISTORY
   Eric Avila
AMERICAN FOREIGN RELATIONS
   Andrew Preston
AMERICAN HISTORY Paul S. Boyer
AMERICAN IMMIGRATION
   David A. Gerber

AMERICAN INTELLECTUAL
   HISTORY
   Jennifer Ratner-Rosenhagen
THE AMERICAN JUDICIAL
   SYSTEM Charles L. Zelden
AMERICAN LEGAL HISTORY
   G. Edward White
AMERICAN MILITARY HISTORY
   Joseph T. Glatthaar
AMERICAN NAVAL HISTORY
   Craig L. Symonds
AMERICAN POETRY David Caplan
AMERICAN POLITICAL HISTORY
   Donald Critchlow
AMERICAN POLITICAL PARTIES
   AND ELECTIONS L. Sandy Maisel
AMERICAN POLITICS
   Richard M. Valelly
THE AMERICAN PRESIDENCY
   Charles O. Jones
THE AMERICAN REVOLUTION
   Robert J. Allison
AMERICAN SLAVERY
   Heather Andrea Williams
THE AMERICAN SOUTH
   Charles Reagan Wilson
THE AMERICAN WEST Stephen Aron
AMERICAN WOMEN'S HISTORY
   Susan Ware
AMPHIBIANS T. S. Kemp
ANAESTHESIA Aidan O'Donnell
ANALYTIC PHILOSOPHY
   Michael Beaney
ANARCHISM Alex Prichard

Available soon:

VATICAN II Shaun Blanchard &
  Stephen Bullivant
OBSERVATIONAL ASTRONOMY
  Geoff Cottrell

MATHEMATICAL ANALYSIS
  Richard Earl
HISTORY OF EMOTIONS
  Thomas Dixon

For more information visit our website

www.oup.com/vsi/

Keith Humphreys

ADDICTION

A Very Short Introduction

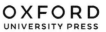
OXFORD
UNIVERSITY PRESS

OXFORD
UNIVERSITY PRESS

Great Clarendon Street, Oxford, OX2 6DP,
United Kingdom

Oxford University Press is a department of the University of Oxford.
It furthers the University's objective of excellence in research, scholarship,
and education by publishing worldwide. Oxford is a registered trade mark of
Oxford University Press in the UK and in certain other countries

First edition published in 2023

Impression: 1

Published in the United States of America by Oxford University Press
198 Madison Avenue, New York, NY 10016, United States of America

British Library Cataloguing in Publication Data
Data available

Library of Congress Control Number: 2022943415

ISBN 978-0-19-955723-3

Printed and bound by
CPI Group (UK) Ltd, Croydon, CR0 4YY

Contents

Preface: the tragedy and mystery of addiction

Imagine hundreds of millions of people in agony. Their health is failing, they are straining to support themselves financially, they are acting in ways that violate their deeply held sense of right and wrong, and they are causing great pain to people whom they love. This describes the population of people who are addicted to drugs, and makes their experience tragic, even heartbreaking. Yet if a fairy godmother appeared and said, "I can take all this pain away by waving my wand and making all drugs disappear from earth," most of the assembled would howl in protest, seize the wand from her hand, and break it in two. That also describes the population of people who are addicted to drugs, and makes their experience mysterious, even maddening.

I have spent the past 35 years trying to understand the tragedy and to unravel the mystery of addiction. This book is an effort to share some of the key things I and my colleagues in the addiction field have learned, as well as to convey the steps that individuals, families, communities, and policymakers can do to lessen the toll of addiction on human health, safety, and well-being.

Acknowledgments

I incurred several debts in writing a VSI to Addiction. Professor Sir John Strang gave valuable advice on what to cover in this slim volume. Ms Ryelee Vest carefully proofread the entire manuscript. A sabbatical grant from Stanford University provided essential writing time. Most importantly, over my career, thousands of people have shared with me their experience of addiction, without which I could never have attained the understanding required to produce this book.

List of illustrations

Chapter 1
Understanding the terrain

Basic terms about drugs and drug use

As with any other complex topic, some definitions are necessary to provide a shared basis of understanding. You do not need to grapple with extensive jargon to understand addiction and to learn from this book, but the following terms are important to know.

Addictive drug. There's an old joke that a drug is defined as any substance that when injected into a laboratory animal results in a peer-reviewed journal article. It sometimes seems that way, but the real definition is that a drug is a chemical substance with a specific molecular structure that when consumed produces a characteristic physiological effect (e.g., wakefulness, sleepiness, agitation, sexual arousal). Consumption of drugs can occur via many routes (see Box: Common methods of consuming drugs).

Human beings of course eat food, drink water, and inhale air, all of which have a particular molecular structure and characteristic physiologic effects. But substances that all human beings must consume to survive are not considered drugs.

Neither are all drugs addictive. People do not become addicted to antibiotics (e.g., penicillin), non-steroidal anti-inflammatory

Common methods of consuming drugs

Swallowing. Alcohol, caffeinated beverages (e.g., coffee, tea), and most prescribed drugs taken as directed are swallowed by the user. Because such drugs are subjected to metabolic processes (e.g., stomach acid breaks them down before they reach the brain) any pharmacologic effects may be delayed relative to other methods of administration.

Within the mouth. The oral cavity is lined with tissue that can absorb drugs. One example will be familiar to fans of American baseball: The wad of tobacco in a player's cheek or the snuff between the cheek and gum provides a steady dose of nicotine. In addition to such "buccal" methods, drugs can also be absorbed sublingually, that is, under the tongue, as is done for example with some formulations (e.g., sprayed, liquefied, or in a film) of opioid medications such as buprenorphine.

Snorting. This method involves inhaling drugs into the nasal cavity where they are rapidly absorbed. Typically, the drug would be in powder form (e.g., powder cocaine) although this method can also work to a limited extent with liquefied drugs such as sprayed naloxone.

Inhalation. Many drugs are consumed by inhaling them in a gaseous form. Most commonly, this is done by heating the drug, often along with other materials, and the smoke being inhaled into the lung. Because of the large surface area of the lung and its absorptive qualities, smoked drugs reach the brain quickly and can thus be highly reinforcing. Tobacco and cannabis cigarettes are the most prevalent examples of a smoked drug ignited by a flame (e.g., a match or lighter), but heroin, crack cocaine, and other drugs also are often smoked. Other ways of inhaling heated nicotine (i.e., e-cigarettes and "heat not burn" cigarettes) do not involve an open flame, but are otherwise similar to smoking as a method of administration. Some people who use drugs inhale products designed for other purposes (e.g., glue, paint thinner, gasoline) to attain intoxicating effects.

Injection. Drugs that are manufactured in liquid form or can be converted to it by users (e.g., through melting a pill or powder) can be injected directly into a vein. This allows the user to rapidly experience the effects of a large amount of a drug. For this reason, individuals who become tolerant to a drug that they have previously taken by swallowing or snorting may cross over to injection use. Injection use likely carries the highest risk of overdose, and certainly has the highest risk of being a vector for the transmission of infectious diseases such as HIV/AIDS, tuberculosis, and various strains of hepatitis.

drugs (e.g., ibuprofen), or antipyretics (e.g., paracetamol), for example. The subset of drugs that are addictive produce a range of short-term, often quite intense effects such as increased happiness, greater energy, reduced anxiety, and lessened pain. Some addictive drugs (e.g., cannabis) also cause alterations in consciousness (e.g., a perception that the pace of time has altered, hearing unusual sounds or voices, thinking in offbeat ways, seeing things that are not there). The short-term effects of addictive drugs differ from the effects they have longer term, which as we will explore can be quite aversive.

When the term drug or addictive drug is mentioned, most people think of crack cocaine, MDMA (also known as ecstasy), and other drugs that are universally illegal. But legally prescribed drugs such as opioids and benzodiazepines are still drugs even though we commonly call them medicines instead. So too are legal recreational drugs like the alcohol (ethanol) in a glass of wine and the nicotine in a combusted or electronic cigarette.

The most widely consumed addictive drugs include ethanol (alcohol), nicotine (mainly in tobacco), and cannabis. Two other widely used classes of drugs are opiates and stimulants. Opiates include opium, morphine, heroin, fentanyl, oxycodone, and hydrocodone. Widely used stimulants include caffeine (coffee), areca nut (also called betel nut), methamphetamine, amphetamine, and cocaine.

Hallucinogens such as LSD, peyote, and psilocybin (the psychoactive component of "magic mushrooms") represent a distinct class of drugs from an addiction viewpoint. Although these are certainly drugs, they do not seem to be particularly addictive. This doesn't mean they aren't ever harmful, only that neither animals nor humans seem to display the signs of addiction that will be described later in this chapter. Such drugs therefore fall outside the scope of this book.

Tolerance. Our bodies adapt to the repeated administration of addictive drugs in multiple ways, one of which is the development of tolerance. Tolerance refers to a drug losing its power to induce an effect at a familiar dose. For example, a person who feels euphoric and relaxed when consuming 20 mg of oxycodone may find that, over time, they need 40 mg to generate the same level of euphoria and relaxation they once felt. And after a period of using 40 mg of oxycodone, the same pattern may repeat, incentivizing the use of ever larger doses.

Tolerance occurs across a range of drug effects. The dose of morphine that eliminated pain from an injury may fail to do so after weeks or months, resulting in "breakthrough pain." The slurred speech and intoxication that followed three pints of beer may not make themselves known until the sixth pint after years of heavy drinking.

Tolerance does not necessarily proceed at the same rate across the effects of the drug. For example, the subjective high from the same dose of an opioid may lessen after fewer uses than does slowed breathing. As a result, someone who increases their dose of opioids to chase the high that has been lost through tolerance may be at unusually high risk of brain damage or death as breathing slows dramatically or even stops because they were not equally tolerant to that effect of the drug.

Tolerance is a natural process within the human brain, and is unique neither to addiction nor drug use. Consider the delight you would feel if you came into the office or a classroom and saw to your surprise that a treat you enjoy, maybe warm chocolate chip cookies or sweet sticky buns, was on offer. But when it turns out that by policy a new tray of the same treat will be there every day to greet you upon arrival, day by day the experience becomes routine and it no longer excites you as it did the first time. The first versus the thousandth time you kiss your sweetheart may be a similar contrast as you acquire tolerance to that reward. So it is with addictive drugs.

Tolerance can also be lost. A person who doesn't use a drug for an extended period will usually find that lower doses have more potent effects than they used to. Some people who are addicted to drugs use this as a conscious strategy, for example by attending a methadone maintenance clinic for a year in the hopes of lowering the amount of heroin they need to get high. Loss of tolerance can also create significant risk. For example, after a period of incarceration during which an individual cannot use drugs, a person may consume their "usual dose" again upon release and find that they lose all inhibitions and do something violent (e.g., with alcohol), or have a health crisis when they pass out suddenly or stop breathing (e.g., with opioids).

Dependence and withdrawal. Just as repeated use of an addictive drug can over time induce tolerance, it can also produce a related but distinct adaptation in the body known as dependence. Dependence means that in the absence of the drug, the person begins to experience withdrawal symptoms which are generally the opposite of the effects of the drug. To cite a common, less severe example, if you regularly drink several cups of coffee at breakfast, a morning without it may leave you feeling unusually sleepy and irritable or perhaps even give you a headache. More aversive examples are that withdrawal from benzodiazepines may be experienced as extreme anxiety, and withdrawal from opioids as agitation, diarrhea, sweats and shakes, sleeplessness, and formication (the disturbing sensation that bugs are crawling under one's skin). Withdrawal from alcohol can involve "delirium tremens" characterized by seizures, high fever, mental confusion, and hallucinations, as well as carrying a risk of death. However, in most cases withdrawal from even heavy drinking, while unpleasant, is less dramatic and dangerous.

Withdrawal is time limited, but some individuals will find it sufficiently unpleasant that they decide to take their drug again, thereby ending the withdrawal symptoms but maintaining their dependence. At one time it was thought that the desire to relieve withdrawal symptoms was the primary cause of relapse. But careful research showed that many addicted people return to substance use long after withdrawal symptoms have faded.

In popular language, people will sometimes make a distinction between "psychological dependence" and "physical dependence" on drugs (e.g., cannabis). But because what we experience as psychological dependence derives from physical structures in the brain, this distinction is scientifically meaningless.

"Overdose." This term is in scare quotes to reflect its deceptive nature. In common parlance as well as sometimes in medicine, the term overdose is used to refer to acute and dangerous effects of addictive drugs. But a more accurate term is "poisoning." The distinction matters because many opioid "overdoses" in fact involve people taking their usual dose or indeed even a lower than normal dose. The same dose can induce poisoning for many reasons, such as loss of ability to metabolize the drug due to age,

the presence of another condition that weakens the person (e.g., flu, exhaustion), or the presence of another drug in the body that produces a dangerous drug–drug interaction. Not acknowledging this can provide a false sense of security, for example that as long as you use the same dose of heroin each day, you will never overdose. But in truth people die every day from taking their usual dose, because heroin at all doses carries a risk of poisoning.

Harm. The term harm is used in the addiction field very much the way "damage" is used outside of it. It refers to the negative consequences of an individual's drug use. These can be consequences for the individual (e.g., waking up in acute withdrawal each day) or for other people (e.g., the employer who loses business because an addicted employee is chronically absent from work). Harms can result from biology (e.g., overdose) or from a social response (e.g., a spouse initiates divorce, a policeman arrests the person for being drunk and disorderly). Importantly, harm exists whether or not the addicted person is aware of it (e.g., undiagnosed liver disease, the loss of respect of one's children, anxiety in one's loved ones). Many people whose addiction damages other people will claim "I am only hurting myself" and genuinely believe this to be true.

Positive and negative reinforcement. Behavioral psychology as formulated by giants like B. F. Skinner is often fairly criticized for oversimplifying human experience. Yet there is still enormous explanatory power in the principle of operant conditioning, namely that the reason human beings do many of the things they do is that they have learned that their behavior produces a desired result. For example, if when you hug your young child your child warmly hugs you back, or laughs and smiles, or says "I love you," you are more likely to hug your child the next day than you are once they are teenagers and they are more likely to respond by stiffening up, protesting that they are too old for hugs, or rolling their eyes.

In the case of drugs, the principle of operant conditioning implies that many people use them because they find the effects of drugs enjoyable. "Enjoyable" is subjective and varies across people, for example one person might find an alteration in consciousness exciting and another person might find it upsetting. But whatever the nature of the specific effect, if it increases the person's likelihood of using the drug again, it is called "reinforcement."

Relative to other forms of reinforcement, that produced by addictive drugs can be extremely powerful. This is in part due to the intensity of reinforcement but also the speed. It takes only a matter of seconds for inhaled cigarette smoke to send nicotine through the lungs, through the blood, and into the brain. The effects of injecting drugs like heroin are also rapid. Human beings are more attuned to immediate rewards than distant ones, and people who are addicted even more so: The immediate pleasure of a smoke right now drives many people's behavior more than avoiding lung cancer that will take decades to develop. The preface of this book pointed out that even people whose lives are being destroyed by addiction still often want drugs, and the intensity and speed of the reinforcement drugs provide is the reason why.

Reinforcement can be positive or negative. Positive reinforcement "adds something" desirable in response to a behavior. For drug use, the burst of energy from using methamphetamine, the mental acuity from consuming nicotine, or the happiness from using opioids, are examples. Quite understandably, whether people are addicted or not, these experiences increase the likelihood of future drug use.

Negative reinforcement "subtracts something" undesirable in response to a behavior. In the case of drugs, this might be the whisky which "takes the edge off" after a hard day, the benzodiazepine which ends a panic attack, or the opioid which soothes the pain from an injury. The legendary author Edgar

Allan Poe, who struggled for years with drug use, described negative reinforcement vividly:

> I have absolutely no pleasure in the stimulants in which I sometimes so madly indulge. It has not been in the pursuit of pleasure that I have periled life and reputation and reason. It has been the desperate attempt to escape from torturing memories, from a sense of insupportable loneliness and a dread of some strange impending doom.

Positive and negative reinforcement can motivate use of the same drug at different points. The expression "the hair of the dog that bit you" refers to someone addressing a hangover by having a drink in the morning. The drinking of the night before was motivated by positive reinforcement—fun, disinhibition, sociability—but the hair of the dog has the different purpose of reducing the misery of a hangover.

When someone regularly uses an addictive drug for many months or years, they can shift from seeking positive reinforcement to desiring negative reinforcement. For example, they can become tolerant to the rewards of their drug use, and their dependence means they go into withdrawal without the drug. The rock and roll singer Cherie Currie vividly described how drug taking eventually felt:

> Even when I took the drugs I realized that this just wasn't fun anymore. The drugs had become a part of my routine. Something to wake me up. Something to help me sleep. Something to calm my nerves. There was a time when I was able to wake up, go to sleep, and have fun without a pill or a line to help me function. These days it felt like I might have a nervous breakdown if I didn't have them.

Addiction. Having defined some basic terms associated with drug use, we come to the most difficult definition of all: what is addiction, the subject of this book? Let's start with the simplest case, which is how scientists define it in animals.

Among the most creative and important studies ever done in the addiction field were conducted by James Olds and Peter Milner in the 1950s. Working at McGill University in Canada, these pioneering neuroscientists showed that rats given targeted electronic brain stimulation in response to a behavior (e.g., pressing a lever in their cage) would aggressively pursue such stimulation even though it was not essential for survival in preference to activities that are, such as consuming food and water. Subsequent researchers showed that similar behavior could be induced by injecting rats with drugs such as cocaine. Once they had been dosed repeatedly, rats would endure significant pain to keep using drugs (e.g., run across an electrified cage to gain access) and consume cocaine in preference to nutritious food even when they were hungry. Addicted rats will also work very hard (e.g., press a lever 2,000 times an hour) to obtain drugs even though it harms them, that is, they burn enormous calories trying to get drugs that have no nutritive value.

In animal research, addiction is defined by these directly observable phenomena: an animal is considered addicted to a drug when it repeatedly endures negative consequences—up to and including death—in its repeated efforts to use that drug.

Matters become more complex when defining addiction in humans. In humans, other data points enter the equation, specifically the ability of people to articulate their own experience. These include reporting things like "I really planned to stop after two shots of vodka, but ended up drinking the whole bottle" and "I find myself thinking about heroin all day long such that I can't focus on anything else" and "I know that my cocaine use is wrecking my marriage, but I keep using it anyway." Addiction in humans also includes choosing not to do other behaviors, for example participating in school, having a job, volunteering in a community (none of this is relevant to lab rats because there is not exactly much to do in a cage).

Addiction in humans includes directly observable phenomena but is not reducible to them. For example, people who are addicted respond to drugs differently from other rewards in ways that can be seen on brain scans. But none of these studies allows a doctor or scientist to point at a brain region with a particular signature and say "There, that is the addiction" as one might say "There, that is the cancerous tumor" on an X-ray or ultrasound, or "You are pregnant" or "You have anemia" using a tested fluid sample. Neither can we use some count of behavior to define a person as addicted, for example saying that anyone who consumes more than X drinks of alcohol, Y shots of heroin, or Z snorts of cocaine must be addicted.

To understand how science and medicine handle situations like this, imagine you are walking through the forest and you see a cluster of flowers growing. You can observe each of their petals, leaves, and stems, but you can't see their roots, so you don't know if they are all coming from one source (e.g., a single bulb, or a single nutrient in the soil) or whether it is just a coincidence that this batch of flowers grow together. You therefore have to make a guess, or what scientists would call a hypothesis, about what you can't see.

Addiction in humans is a hypothesis that a group of things we can observe have an underlying connection, much as there might be a connection under the soil between a group of flowers we can observe above ground. The most important of those observables, just as in animals, is the repeated use of addictive drugs in the face of harm. It also includes people reporting on experiences such as having their "mental real estate" consumed by drug use, experiencing struggles with control over their use, consuming more than intended (e.g., "I'll just do one line of cocaine" turning into a weekend long binge), and experiencing dependence, tolerance, and withdrawal. Individually none of these things is addiction, but to speak of addiction is to believe they constitute a syndrome. Syndrome literally means "running together." To say that all these observables are a syndrome is to hypothesize that they run together for an underlying reason, which we are calling addiction.

It's useful to revisit the terms laid out in the prior section as they relate to addiction. Tolerance, dependence, and withdrawal are experienced by almost all people who are addicted, but they are not in themselves addiction. You may find that a single glass of wine doesn't reduce anxiety the way it used to because you have become tolerant to the effects of alcohol, but that doesn't necessarily mean that you are experiencing harm or that you struggle to control your drinking. Dependence is often falsely equated with addiction, and this was not helped by medical nomenclature in the past using them interchangeably. But many people who take opioids for pain for weeks or longer will experience withdrawal when they quit yet not go on to use opioids in an addictive fashion. Instead the withdrawal fades with time and they do not use opioids any more.

Not all harmful substance use is addiction either. Someone who hardly ever drinks can get intoxicated at the office holiday party and then get a ticket for driving erratically on the way home, but this doesn't mean they are addicted to alcohol. Indeed, even someone who engages in harmful substance use on multiple occasions is not necessarily addicted. The latest editions of the International Classification of Diseases (ICD) and Diagnostic and Statistical Manual of Mental Disorders (DSM) recognize this by allowing clinicians to record harmful substance use that does not rise to the level of addiction, even though neither uses this term. Most people whom the ICD deems as "substance dependent" would be considered addicted as would most people whom the DSM diagnoses as being at the "severe" end of what it calls "substance use disorder."

At the same time, harm is essential to the definition of addiction. We speak colloquially of "being addicted to" many activities that we engage in repeatedly, whether it's listening to jazz music, shopping for handbags, checking our email, collecting rare coins, or playing a particular video game. But simply engaging in a behavior much more than other people and thinking about it often is not inherently proof of an addiction. Unless the behavior is genuinely causing harm, for example a person bankrupts themselves buying handbags or stops eating and sleeping and showing up for work in order to play a video game, there is no reason to invoke addiction as an explanation.

Chapter 2
The nature of addiction

The first chapter defined addiction as a syndrome—is it also a disease? This is a much debated issue about which there is more heat than light. A key reason for this is that the word disease is used in markedly different ways by different people.

The founders of Alcoholics Anonymous and the 12-step movement it spawned call addiction a disease. But they don't mean disease in a biomedical sense, defining it instead as something rooted in a person's character (e.g., self-centeredness) and having physical, psychological, and spiritual components. From the point of view of the 12-step disease model, recovery requires cessation of substance use but also more than that, namely reconstruction of moral character coupled with spiritual growth.

A different disease model, propagated mainly by the US National Institutes on Health, is that addiction is a "brain disease," specifically that repeated consumption of addictive drugs alters brain structure, pathways, and functioning in adverse ways. This disease model emphatically rules out considerations of moral character, being entirely biological. The brain disease model maintains that repeated consumption of drugs can cause neural adaptations that could be thought of as a form of deeply maladaptive learning. Behaviors focused on obtaining and using drugs become entrenched through reinforcement. The neurotransmitter-based motivational system of the brain becomes distorted such that natural rewards become increasingly less appealing relative to drugs. The part of the brain that normally helps us restrain our impulses functions less well. To the addicted person, this can feel as if the gas pedal is sticking to the floor and the brakes are failing at the same time.

There is also evidence that other parts of the brain change such that the person's "emotional set point" moves downward, creating a sense of pervasive unease. This makes long-term drug use as much about relief from negative feelings and "trying to get back to where I started" as it is about attaining an elevated mood state. At the risk of oversimplifying, imagine that our mood could be judged on a 1–10 scale at any given moment with 10 being the most wonderful and 1 the most miserable. An addicted person who once woke up with a mood score of 5 each day and used drugs to reach a score of 10 may start waking up at 1 and need drugs just to return to the 5 that was once their set point.

Yet another framing of addiction is as a bad habit, that is, that a person is repeatedly engaging in activity that damages their health, much as does overeating which leads to obesity. This model assumes that like other well-entrenched behaviors, addictive behavior is hard to change. Individuals embracing this viewpoint usually don't explicitly describe addiction as a disease, being more likely to describe it as a chronic health problem, complex behavioral disorder, or a behavioral health problem.

Although people who describe addiction in terms of behavior, learning, and environmental responses tend to reject the "brain disease" model as too reductionist, too American, or both, this does not mean they think the brain is irrelevant. After all, the brain is where memories of learned associations are stored and also clearly affects human behavior. To wit, the Scottish naval physician Thomas Trotter, who in 1804 wrote the first English-language book on alcohol addiction and its treatment, emphasized the role of habit in the maintenance of what he called "drunkenness." Yet he also famously wrote "the habit of drunkenness is a disease of the mind."

The differences between various models of addiction aside, all of them view addiction as a chronic challenge rather than an acute one. An infection, a broken bone, a bruise, and many other health problems are short term in nature, healing on their own or with time-limited medical intervention. But addiction is a long-term problem. From the 12-step disease conception, it can be arrested but never cured. The brain disease model is more optimistic that addiction can be cured in at least some cases (particularly with a young person) but certainly views recovery as a long-term process requiring long-term support. And those who see it as a behavioral health problem also recognize that changing behavior in a lasting fashion is difficult and typically requires extended support and effort.

Whether people call addiction a disease rather than for example a sin or a character flaw commonly reflects their views on how society should respond to it, that is, with rage versus compassion, blame versus forgiveness, punishment versus assistance. So for example, someone might endorse the brain disease model because they think that relative to defining addiction as a sin it will make the public and policymakers more sympathetic towards addicted people. Someone else, who lost a family member to an intoxicated driver, may say addiction cannot be a disease because the person who killed their loved one deserves punishment and we don't typically punish people for having a disease. But of course whether a belief has a particular consequence for the person who holds it or anyone else is a distinct question from whether or not it is factually accurate: Believing that you can fly may be exciting, even thrilling, but it does not mean you should try it when next you are on top of a tall building.

Rather than use arguments about whether addiction is a disease as proxies for questions about responsibility and blame, let's take on such questions directly.

Isn't heavy substance use simply willful misconduct? Beer doesn't leap into our mouths. Heroin doesn't melt itself and climb into a syringe that then forcefully injects the drug into our veins. Substance use is a behavior in which people choose to engage. All of us are responsible for the decisions we make, including our decisions to use substances and to use them to the point of intoxication.

That is where we all start in life, but is it still true of the subset of people whose chosen substance use results in them becoming addicted? Some view addiction as a Rubicon in which all control is lost, meaning that the disease completely robs people of agency and therefore any responsibility for their conduct. But the evidence suggests it is not that simple. Even pack a day smokers will refrain from smoking in certain circumstances (e.g., on holy days if they are religious) and even people addicted to alcohol lessen their consumption in response to tax increases. More generally, there are hundreds of millions of people in the world who have recovered from addiction, which would be impossible if addiction eliminated human agency. Perhaps some people do lose all self-control during addiction, for example through brain damage, but were that the norm, recovery would be exceedingly rare, which it is not.

To say that most people retain self-control during addiction is not equivalent to saying their self-control is unimpaired. Abstaining from drug use or using drugs in moderate amounts is harder for someone who is addicted, because their desire to use is stronger and the ability to resist urges is weaker than that experienced by non-addicted people. Here is an analogy: Two people are each handed a glass of cool, delicious, lemonade, but told not to drink it. Only one of the two people has just spent a day walking in the desert. Both people are capable of refraining from drinking, but the effort needed to do so is much greater for the desert walker, and we should be more sympathetic to that person if they cannot do it than to the person who hadn't had that experience.

Is it unfair to be angry at addicted people who have harmed you? Sometimes the addiction as a brain disease model is presented in a scolding fashion that feels like a put down to people who feel hurt and angry about something that an addicted person in their life did, that is, "If you were just smart enough to understand neuroscience, you would know that you shouldn't be angry at someone for having a disease!" Discounting people's suffering just because the person who inflicted it had impaired control is wrong-headed and sometimes even cruel, because it ignores how many people have been genuinely harmed by the conduct of people during addiction. Being angry, hurt, distressed, and frightened is a natural human reaction to being victimized, whether the perpetrator was addicted or not. To discount those feelings on the assumption that a rational person should be able to fully control their reactions in light of the brain disease of addiction is internally contradictory: it emphasizes the limits of control over behavior and affect for addicted people, without extending that understanding to the rest of humanity. Just as it may be hard for a father who is addicted to alcohol not to get drunk at his teenaged daughter's birthday party even though he rationally knows he should not drink, it is hard for his daughter not to feel humiliated by his behavior even if she rationally knows her father has limited self-control because of his addiction.

Can addicted people reasonably blame the environment for their behavior? One despairing view of addiction considers it a self-contained phenomenon—the person is completely out of control, which is sad, but cannot be helped. But the truth is that even severely addicted people respond to their environment, for example how available drugs are, the cues to use them (e.g., advertising), what they cost, how approving or disapproving friends and family are, and the like. Further, the environment of one's family and community shapes a person's risk of becoming addicted and another environmental feature—the availability of supports for recovery—influences a person's likelihood of recovering from addiction. No addiction is an island. Individual effort certainly matters but the initiation, course, and severity of an addiction is determined in part by the environment.

On that note, a common critique of the idea of addiction as a brain disease is that it rules out public health interventions by locating the problem between the ears of the addicted person. But brains don't float in the ether; they are inherently shaped by environment. So there is nothing inconsistent in believing that the brain matters in addiction while trying to change the environment around it.

"Behavioral" addiction

Most of this book has focused on addiction to drugs like alcohol, nicotine, cannabis, and cocaine. But does it end there? Should it? The most recent editions of the US Diagnostic and Statistical Manual of Mental Disorders (DSM) and the International Classification of Diseases (ICD) include "gambling disorder" as an established diagnosis. The former also includes "Internet gaming disorder" as a condition meriting further study and the latter includes "gaming disorder" as an established diagnosis in a category called "Disorders due to addictive behavior." The criteria for both conditions mention phenomena often seen in people addicted to drugs, including tolerance, subjective loss of control, continued engagement in addictive behavior despite harm, and extensive time spent engaging in the behavior and thinking about it. There has also been significant advocacy inside and outside of psychiatry to define a range of sexual behaviors as addictions in future editions of the DSM.

Beyond the halls of medicine, in daily life, people speak of addiction to a broad range of activities: "I'm totally hooked on EastEnders," "I'm addicted to Twitter," "I need my daily fix of World of Warcraft," "I left my iPhone at home today and I'm in withdrawal," "I am completely craving chocolate ice cream." Are they referring to a phenomenon that is analogous to the experience of the chain-smoker or the person who injects himself with heroin every eight hours?

Widening or narrowing the definition of addiction is not just a theoretical debate, but a decision with real-world consequences. Some of the consequences are political. For example, governments spend money on addiction treatment. If the definition of addiction is broadened, governments might be pressured to spend more on treatment, or they might spread the existing money over more people, lessening the quality of care for all.

In law, expanding the definition of addiction might have positive or negative implications for whether we hold people responsible for their conduct. A number of famous serial sexual harassers have announced in the press that they are entering rehab for their sexual addiction. Will that mean that they evade punishment and will no longer fear to continue their behavior? Alternatively, would defining as addicted someone who is sexually aroused by women's shoes and repeatedly shoplifts them for erotic pleasure help them avoid a harsh punishment they don't deserve and instead justify directing them to treatment?

Other consequences are cultural. A collective decision that, say, someone who loses all his money on electronic slot machines is addicted may bring that person sympathy and help. On the other hand, because addiction is a stigmatized condition, broadening its definition could tarnish the reputation of harmless people or activities. Someone who is happy spending every spare penny on his stamp collection and who spends eight hours a day thinking about, reading about, and seeking out stamps may be angered that the life he finds fulfilling is labelled as a disease or sin.

A particular concern in this area centers on sexual behavior. It was literally chapter and verse in psychiatric medicine 50 years ago (i.e., in the DSM) that homosexuality was a diagnosable disease, a case where the field was no doubt influenced by reigning morals regarding sex. Given how comfortable many people are judging the sexuality of others, and the demonstrated potential of those judgments to seep into what should be a scientifically grounded field, particular caution must be exercised to not label uncommon sources of sexual gratification as addictions simply because they offend present-day sensibilities.

The consequence of defining things as diseases is an independent consideration of whether they really are diseases. Empirical concerns exist regarding whether many non-drug-related behaviors can be called addictions. Some people who gamble away their life savings feel all the same emotions as do people who squander their life savings on cocaine: Loss of control, emotional high points followed by despair, compulsive urges and thoughts, and the like. But that doesn't mean objectively that the two situations are the same. A torn intercostal muscle in the right location creates for the person who experiences it tightness in the chest, difficulty breathing, pain, and numbness. It may therefore feel to the person concerned terrifyingly like a heart attack. But it's not a heart attack and should not be treated as such in any sense of the word "treated."

As laid out in Chapter 1, we are handicapped here because addiction is a syndrome that we do not observe directly but infer from things we can observe directly such as repeated use despite harm, tolerance, and withdrawal. For that reason, we cannot be completely sure whether somewhere inside the brain of the person who spends 20 hours a day playing internet games as their life and health disintegrate is the root of a disorder that is the same as someone who does the same with drinking alcohol.

The argument on whether behavioral addictions are indeed addictions thus must be waged over the observables we have.

The one that leaps out as most informative is harm. When harm is taken into account, many common references to "being addicted" to something are clearly not addiction. Perhaps someone has died from using Twitter too much, for example because they tweeted while driving their car and ran into a tree, but that can't compare to the chance of dying from smoking, which about one-third of tobacco addicted people will do. Surely some fans feel powerful urges to watch their favorite television show, but there have been few if any people who lost their job, health, and family because of it. And although it's hard to find people who inject heroin several times a day and are at the same time healthy, happy, and productive, it's easy to find people who check their iPhone 300 times a day and are all of these things.

If we bear the standard of harm in mind, we are left with a much shorter list of behaviors that might be called addictions, and even then mainly at the extreme end. One is gambling. A subset of individuals who gamble experience massive harms, not only financial but also from neglect of their families and friends and also their health. The anthropologist Natasha Dow Schüll documented some individuals compulsively playing slot machines in adult diapers so that they can urinate and defecate in place without the need of a bathroom break. Schüll also describes a scene captured on a casino camera in which a player had a cardiac arrest and fell to the floor, and none of the other gamblers even hesitated to continue playing around him.

A critic of the proposition that gambling is an addiction might note that smoking and drinking while gambling is extremely common and perhaps the gambling is merely learnt through the associated reinforcement of drugs. But some gamblers do not use addictive substances yet still find gambling independently addictive.

At a policy level, another similarity of gambling to other addictions is that an industry makes enormous profits from it, and has learned how to make their product ever more addictive. As with alcohol, tobacco, and other drugs, pushing back on the problem requires not just help for individuals but also tighter controls on ruthless corporate profit seeking.

Computer gaming may also be considered an addiction in some extreme cases. Extensive media attention has focused on unmarried, young males who have mediocre jobs, live in their parents' basement, and play video games with each other all day. But these same journalistic accounts generally report that these individuals are having a great deal of fun and it is not clear that they are damaging themselves or anyone else even though many people on the outside might describe their life as unappealing or disreputable. That said, the very rare cases of adolescents engaging in violence or self-harm when their parents restrict their video game access or collapsing after 18 or more hours straight of gaming may be appropriate to understand in the terms of addiction.

Sexual addictions seem in some respects an even closer potential analogy to some substance focused addictions. Orgasm produces a chemical, ecstatic rush including endogenous opioid release. Some people also seem to experience tolerance to sexual experiences. For example, a fantasy of being seen masturbating is initially rewarding but then becomes routine, leading the person to go through the same cycle of reward and tolerance with progressively more extreme behaviors (e.g., actually masturbating in a park away from people, intentionally doing so within sight of them, and then exposing oneself in situations where being seen is a certainty).

However, terming sexual behavior addiction does run into a conceptual problem insofar as sex is an evolved behavior essential to pass on genes and hence naturally pleasurable. We could never logically ask, "What disaster befell this person such that they enjoy sex?" or "The best prevention and treatment is lifetime abstinence." If human beings stopped consuming tobacco, heroin, and cocaine, and never went to another slot machine, our collective health and safety would be enhanced as would that of future generations. But without sex, humans would die out, so eliminating it would ensure harm rather than forestalling it.

This problem becomes even more pronounced with the questionable concept of "food addiction." Human beings must have sex to create the next generation; they must eat from their first day on earth for the survival of their own. Food keeps us alive and not eating soon kills us, so any effort to establish the harm of "food addiction" will come to no good.

A more "refined" definition is that human beings can become addicted to sugar and high fat foods. Here again we are stretching the usual definition of addiction in that for most of our evolutionary heritage food supply was lower and those who were able to access high calorie foods were more evolutionarily fit. What has changed isn't our taste for such foods, but agriculture and the modern food industry. We of course may like foods that are not good for us in the long term, so that we would be healthier if we ate less of them, but none of that need bring in the concept of addiction.

The prevalence of addiction

Determining how many people are addicted is challenging because different studies in different countries use different criteria, and indeed even within countries the criteria change over time as diagnostic systems are revised. Holding those grains of salt in mind, epidemiological surveys can give at least some sense of the prevalence of addiction.

In the United States, the federal government conducts a large sample annual survey of the population aged 12 and older. It does not include individuals who are incarcerated or who live on the street (though it does include people in homeless shelters) and thus should be assumed to understate addiction even if one assumed that people who are surveyed had no reticence about disclosing. That said, it found that 60.1 percent of Americans over the age of 12 (165 million people) used at least one psychoactive substance in the past month. About one-eighth of those individuals (about 7.5 percent of the population or 20.4 million) met criteria for a substance use disorder other than tobacco. Of those individuals, 71.1 percent had an alcohol use disorder, 40.7 percent had an illicit drug use disorder, and 11.8 percent had both. The survey found that about 27 million people were daily cigarette smokers, almost all of whom were likely addicted, and many of whom would also have other substance use disorders as well. A different US study known as NESARC generated similar but slightly higher estimated prevalence of "alcohol abuse or dependence" (8.5 percent) and "illicit drug abuse or dependence" (2.0 percent), which were the diagnostic terms at the time. These results are similar to what has been found in studies of the European Union as a whole, though individual countries vary in the prevalence of addiction.

The United Kingdom conducts standing surveys only of some addictions. About 15 percent of British adults smoke cigarettes, and high rates of addiction in this group are suggested by about a third smoking within 30 minutes of waking up in the morning and almost two-thirds expressing a desire to quit. England conducts a national survey of the prevalence of gambling disorder, which is experienced by 0.7 percent of the adult population. About 1.5 percent of the English adult population is estimated to have a serious enough alcohol problem to warrant treatment; the proportion who at least occasionally binge drink is at least 10 times that high. Illicit drug use data is gathered in the British Crime Survey (which only covers England and Wales). Over 9 percent of individuals aged 16 to 59 used an illicit drug in the past 12 months, but only 2.1 percent used illicit drugs frequently, meaning somewhere between more than once a month to every day.

Studies of the current prevalence of addiction understate how many people will be affected at one time or another. Epidemiological studies that also examine lifetime prevalence typically find it is 2–3 times higher than current prevalence. Over 9 percent of American adults say they at one point had a serious alcohol or drug problem and now no longer do, providing converging support for the idea that at any given time the proportion of the adult population who is either currently or formerly addicted ranges between one-sixth and a fourth.

Many people assume that because poverty correlates with worse health, the rates of addiction described above for the United States and Europe would be much lower than what is experienced in low income countries. But the reverse is true: Low income countries tend to have lower rates of addiction than middle and high income countries. When low income countries develop economically, their addiction rates tend to rise, as has been seen for example in South Africa, Brazil, and India (Figure 1).

Studies of the prevalence of substance use disorders vary in methods and historical era, but still suggest some important general lessons. Addiction is in fact a common condition, albeit one that may be hidden from public view. Even with all the ways that surveys undercount the prevalence of addiction, studies across countries and eras show that about 1 in 12 people is addicted to alcohol or illicit drugs, and this figure does not include people addicted to tobacco or to gambling. Studies also show consistently that the proportion of people who have an addiction in the past or will develop one in the future is even larger than those currently affected. By extension, even most people who will never experience addiction themselves will know someone and likely multiple people in their lives, for example, in their families, friendship circles, at school or at work, who currently or in the past experienced addiction.

Share of the population with alcohol or drug use disorders, 2019

Alcohol or drug use dependence is defined by the International Classification of Diseases as the presence of three or more indicators of dependence for at least a month within the previous year.

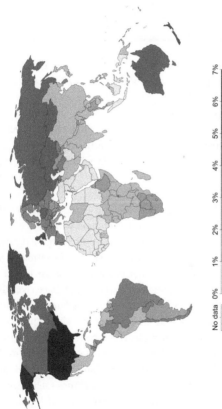

No data 0% 1% 2% 3% 4% 5% 6% 7%

Source: IHME, Global Burden of Disease (2019)

Note: Tobacco smoking is not included. Due to the widespread under-diagnosis, these estimates use a combination of sources, including medical and national records, epidemiological data, survey data, and meta-regression models.

OurWorldInData.org/substance-use • CC BY

1. Low income countries have the lowest rates of addiction.

The effects of addiction

Describing the effect of a fractured collar bone or the common cold is fairly straightforward. But because addiction alters the consciousness of the person who experiences it, changes relationships with other people, and can have radiating effects on community safety, its effects require more elaboration across these domains.

Experientially, addiction can be all-encompassing, shaping behavior, self-perceptions, moods, and interactions with others. Family members, friends, goals, and activities that were once central to a person's life are neglected as the person engages in a full-time quest to seek and use the drug or drugs to which they are addicted. Attention and thought once allocated over a wide range of activities narrows to focus on when, where, and how drugs can be obtained and used.

For other individuals, addiction may coexist with other priorities and responsibilities. This is most common with tobacco but sometimes occurs with other drugs as well, with the person using drugs in a health damaging fashion while still continuing to function for many years, sometimes at an impressive level. Winston Churchill's prodigious alcohol and tobacco consumption (he was surely addicted to the latter and perhaps the former as well) is a famous example. Many more prosaic examples exist, such as the skilled teacher who needs benzodiazepines prior to lecturing and to get to sleep and amphetamines in the morning to wake up, or the carpenter who works hard all week and then blows almost all of his wages on slot machines each weekend while still managing to squeak by financially. Life's equilibrium in such cases is often fragile, and a change in life context or drug use, or a bit of bad luck, can produce a crisis with damaging consequences that also might stimulate an effort to change.

Most addicted people did not intend or expect to become addicted. A college student describes herself as a social smoker and only uses cigarettes at parties until one day she buys a pack to smoke while writing a term paper, beginning what becomes a daily habit. The construction worker who begins having a few drinks after work finds himself after a decade having a few drinks before work, and then a few more instead of work. Each step in the process feels small, but over time a long journey has been taken, and the person may reflect in shock, "How on earth did it come to this?"

Other people drift in and out of addiction rather than following a linear progression. A woman who uses cocaine almost daily finds the behavior unthinkable once she becomes pregnant and so goes cold turkey. Yet when her children grow up and leave home, she starts dabbling again in drugs during a period of boredom and lack of life direction, and is soon as deeply enmeshed in cocaine addiction as ever.

Taking drugs can be intensely pleasurable and rewarding, particularly in the short term. Some people describe their first use of heroin as "the ultimate warm and cozy blanket in which to wrap myself up" or "the filling of a hole in my spirit that had been there my whole life." Cocaine, methamphetamine, and other stimulant use can make people feel powerful, successful, charismatic, and sexy. Yet the lives of addicted people are usually characterized by miserable experiences as well, particularly as their drug use career progresses. The cannabis-induced stumble down the stairs that leaves painful bruises or fractures a bone, the uncontrollable nosebleeds from chronic cocaine snorting, the hacking morning cough of the cigarette smoker, the splitting headache and nausea of an alcohol hangover, the jittery gloom when the ever-shorter high from heroin starts to fade.

Part of the misery of addiction comes from being unable to accomplish things that once brought pride, meaning, and other rewards. As ability to control one's cravings and use becomes impaired, a once solid student finds that he can no longer focus on doing well on exams even in his favorite courses; the once successful small business owner mismanages things to the point of bankruptcy; a professional athlete sees her performance decay to an amateur level; a dedicated parent becomes volatile and impatient to the point of scaring his or her children. The recognition throughout these humiliations and setbacks that one no longer has full control of one's thoughts, behavior, and life can itself inspire further fear and embarrassment. As the Australian novelist Luke Davies put it, "When you can stop you don't want to, and when you want to stop, you can't…"

One of the most dehumanizing aspects of addiction is how it can lead to people hurting those about whom they care most. To purchase drugs, a mother steals the money that her son has been saving to buy a football. Under the influence of opioids, a father passes out while driving his children to school. During methamphetamine intoxication, someone loses their temper over nothing and physically assaults their best friend. These sorts of incidents often become a source of guilt and shame in the addicted person, and more hurt, anger, and fear in those around them.

As alluded to in the Preface, ambivalence is a common experience in addiction. Even as the damage of substance use piles up, the use itself can still provide intense short-term positive or negative reinforcement. The natural human tendency to value small, immediate rewards over larger but delayed rewards is amplified by addiction. Even though recovery would bring more enduring pleasure, it takes significant time and work to achieve, and thus the experience of resolving to change and then returning to substance use after a few weeks or days or even hours is common. The average person who succeeds at quitting smoking has tried six times before. To be addicted can often mean subjectively hating a drug but also loving it at the same time.

Morbidity and mortality are prevalent consequences of addiction. Use of addictive drugs contributes to about one in six deaths among adults worldwide, and these deaths are concentrated in although not exclusive to addicted individuals. The biggest cause of death is tobacco addiction, which causes premature mortality in almost 8 million people a year globally. Alcohol is the next most deadly drug with about 3 million global deaths annually; this includes a significant number of non-addicted people. Because they are illicit and therefore less widely used, all illicit drugs together cause "only" about 750 million deaths annually. By way of comparison deaths from tobacco, alcohol, and illicit drugs exceed those from all cancers combined.

Average years of life lost by the individual user is another useful metric for understanding the health damage wrought by addiction. Data comes from wildly different samples and should therefore be viewed as estimates, but heroin addiction results in a loss of a quarter-century of life relative to the average for the population, and methamphetamine addiction takes a similar toll. Years of life lost are less, but still significant for other drugs, probably a decade for tobacco addiction and something similar for alcohol addiction. Because polydrug addiction is common, even the preceding ghastly statistics understate the loss of life for many individuals experiencing addiction.

The types of deaths experienced vary. The most direct route is poisoning, otherwise known as overdose. Most addictive drugs increase risks of accidents (e.g., automobile crashes) and a subset (e.g., cocaine, alcohol) increases risk of involvement in violent encounters. Rates of suicide are also elevated in almost all addictions. Other mortality risks become evident more slowly. Multiple addictive drugs, including tobacco, alcohol, and perhaps some opioids, are carcinogenic. Most addictive drugs put acute and chronic strains on the cardiovascular system, raising risk of heart attacks and strokes.

Looking just at deaths actually understates the damage of addiction because so many people live for years with disability: the cocaine-induced stroke that causes left-side paralysis, blindness from drinking methyl alcohol in a desperate effort to stave off withdrawal, hepatitis from sharing injection equipment, brain damage from oxygen deprivation during a non-fatal overdose on opioids. Drugs can also reduce quality of life in less dramatic but significantly impairing ways, for example cannabis addiction reducing concentration, memory, and motivation to the point that someone cannot graduate from school or hold down an intellectually complex job.

Unsurprisingly given the powerful effects of drugs on the brain, the most prevalent morbidities among addicted individuals are psychiatric in nature. Both community and clinical survey studies commonly find that at least half of addictions co-occur with a psychiatric illness. Differentiating the two can be challenging. Indeed, there is a clinical maxim in psychiatry that addiction "can look like anything else": heavy drinking and benzodiazepine use can induce depressed mood and suicidal impulses, stimulant use can amplify anxiety and aggression, and multiple drugs can induce psychotic episodes. Most of these substance-induced psychiatric disorders disappear or at least lessen in severity with abstinence, but not all of them. Most notably, heavy use of potent cannabis in adolescence and young adulthood as well as chronic stimulant use (e.g., of methamphetamine) at any age carry some risk of permanent psychotic illness (e.g., schizophrenia). Whether all or only some drug users are vulnerable to such effects is currently an area of active scholarly investigation and debate.

The link between addiction and other health harm comes about through multiple routes. First, repeated exposure of the body to the substance itself can do damage directly, as in the case of alcohol causing cirrhosis of the liver or tobacco smoking causing lung cancer. Other problems can come from route of drug use, for example hepatitis, HIV/AIDS, or tuberculosis being transmitted through shared drug injection equipment. Still others may be due to intoxication, for example benzodiazepines leading someone to have an accident on the job and thereby suffer an injury, or a person intoxicated on alcohol and MDMA not practicing safe sex as they normally would and thereby contracting a sexually transmitted disease.

Adding up all of the harms of addiction to health and well-being would be very difficult. But regardless of the research method used to make the assessment, addiction is one of the most prevalent causes of morbidity and mortality facing humanity.

Unlike many other common health problems (e.g., hypertension, influenza, asthma) addiction also often has enduring and profound effects on the individual's relationships with others. Addiction can be a maddening experience for the person affected, and perhaps even more so for those who care about them. Part of the suffering people experience can be due to the addicted individual's conduct towards them, which can be seriously harmful in some cases (e.g., intoxicated aggression, driving impaired with a family on board, cancer from second-hand smoke) but is more commonly things such as reduced attention, presence, and time. There may also be occasions of painful embarrassment or shame, for example having to convince a drunken spouse who is making a scene to leave a party, or a child coming home with friends to find a parent drug-impaired. Significant others may often find themselves making excuses for or covering the responsibilities of their addicted loved one.

Great worry about the person who is addicted and frustration at being unable to make them stop are common burdens. Even if the addiction is one that does not produce great disruptions in family life, such as cigarette addiction, it can create worry in others about the health of their loved one, as well as a sense of confusion as to why the person continues to harm their health.

The addicted person's internal world may have changed to the point that it seems impossible that another person could understand them: "…who could agree with someone who was so certain you were going to be sober the day after tomorrow?" says an alcohol-addicted character in Malcolm Lowry's *Under the Volcano*. This can further emotional distance in a relationship.

There was a fashion in pop psychology in the 1980s and 1990s to define everyone who was in a relationship with an addicted individual as a "codependent," often with some element of blame or pathologization attached. However, studies of wives whose husbands were actively addicted to alcohol showed that when the husband entered recovery, the wives' mental health looked the same as those of never-addicted spouses, suggesting that their "codependence" was a reaction to the disorder, not a precipitator of it. As studies by the British psychologist Jim Orford and colleagues have shown, most of the things people in relationship with addicted individuals do—beg for change, worry, cajole, cover up—are signs not of codependent personality but of something more basic: Their love for them.

Impact on public safety

Addiction is a threat to public safety as well as public health, and this must be accounted for in assessing its harm. In a widely cited and influential scientific article, a group of prominent researchers likened addictions to other chronic medical disorders such as hypertension, asthma, and Type II diabetes. In several respects the analogy was apt. All these disorders involve at least some voluntary behavior, and also usually have a chronic course. Further, risk for all these disorders can be transmitted genetically.

However, the analogy of addiction to conditions such as hypertension breaks down when one considers what economists call "negative externalities." People with hypertension are not prone to violence; people with asthma do not steal money; people with Type II diabetes do not kill many thousands of people a year while driving recklessly. But all these negative externalities inflicted on others are common in addiction. In the important sense of having massive public safety impacts, addiction really isn't like those chronic medical disorders.

Addiction is in this respect more like infectious diseases which pose public safety risks, which therefore brings other agencies, such as law enforcement, into play. The classic example is Mary Mallon, who refused to believe that she had typhoid and therefore continued to spread the disease. Eventually, "Typhoid Mary" was arrested by the police and put in involuntary quarantine to protect the public.

Although it is fashionable in some corners to assert that the inherent role of law enforcement in society's response to drug addiction is the fault of "The War on Drugs" making drugs illegal, the biggest culprit is completely legal: alcohol. The British Crime Survey, for example, consistently finds that about three-quarters of all violent incidents that occur between 6 p.m. in the evening and 6 a.m. in the morning involve alcohol. Globally, legal alcohol is involved in a large proportion of murders, assaults, vehicular homicides, etc. and accounts for more arrests and incarceration than all illegal drugs combined. This underscores an important reality that would not change even if more drugs were legalized: most arrests of people who use drugs are not for drug use per se, but for conduct engaged in while using or obtaining drugs.

These and other public safety harms are why there will always be significant interaction between the criminal justice system and people who are addicted, whether drugs are legal or illegal. It also should serve as a reminder that negative feelings about addiction cannot always be dismissed as stigma or lack of comprehension of the nature of addiction, but can stem from understandable hurt, anger, and fear after being victimized.

Chapter 3
Causes of addiction

In trying to understand "What causes addiction?," it helps to consider how that question is directed. Scientists are mainly interested in what causes addiction in general, but non-scientists are often more interested in questions like "Why was my mother addicted to Valium?" or "Why can't I stop taking opioid painkillers?" or "Is there anything I can do to stop my son from being addicted to alcohol and cannabis?"

Science has a great deal to offer about the general question of what causes addiction, but at best can only partly answer questions about the cause of any particular individual's addiction. That is, if someone asks "Why me?" a scientist could point out characteristics the person has that are known to raise risk for addiction, but cannot definitively answer why that particular person is addicted because of the complex and unique ways in which lives and addiction proceed. For example, there are genetic components to addiction, and people with many relatives with addiction are at higher risk in general, but that doesn't prove a specific person who is addicted and had genetic risks would not have become so without those risks; they might have become addicted anyway. And that same addicted person could have an identical twin with the same genes who isn't addicted. Indeed, any given individual could have every risk factor that scientists have identified as contributing to addiction in general, yet avoid the problem.

This may be a bit frustrating to anyone seeking to explain a particular case of addiction, but it doesn't mean the science isn't important, just that it is more useful for other purposes. For example, if we know what raises risk for addiction in general across a population, scientists can help design policies that will on average reduce the rate of addiction even though they will not be able to specify in advance which specific individuals will benefit.

The other conceptual point to consider when asking what causes addiction—without getting too philosophically lofty—is what we mean by "cause." Sometimes people use cause to mean something that contributes to a particular outcome, but at other times people mean it in the sense of "but for," that is, without this element the addiction would never have happened. There is only one "but for" element regarding addiction to a drug, namely that human beings use it. People only get addicted to the drugs they use, and they of course can only use drugs that are available to them. There was no cocaine addiction in all of human history before 1859 because the drug didn't exist, so no one could use it. Similarly, a population or individual who chooses not to use an available drug has no chance of becoming addicted to it. Every other variable science identifies is more probabilistic, something that raises or lowers likelihood of addiction but does not rule it in or out.

So if we are trying to determine why addiction is a prevalent problem for modern humanity, the simplest answer is because there are an enormous number of drugs that humans like and choose to take. To understand how humanity got to this point, consider something old and something new.

Something old: human evolution

If you went back in time a few million years and were asked to place a bet on which creatures would have surviving descendants in the 21st century, you would probably not have plumped for hominins. They could not fly, nor even run particularly fast. Their bodies did not have armored plates, terrifying fangs, or deadly claws. They were not intimidatingly big or strong. Yet they did persist for a different reason: they could learn, plan, and think at a level that now-extinct species couldn't match.

Although smaller than those possessed by modern humans, the brain of early hominins allowed them to form memories, to think ahead, and to learn associations. These associations were formed as human ancestors explored the environment and learned to make behavioral choices, for example to consume one fruit versus another, drink one liquid versus another, or mate with one nice hominin boy or girl versus another. Hominins thus learned and encoded important lessons about the environment that contributed to survival, for example how to get warm when cold, what to eat when hungry, what to drink when thirsty, and how to find a fun date.

For several million years, the lives of hominins and their descendent species were nasty, brutish, and short, because essentials such as nutritious food and physical safety were often scarce. Being highly motivated to seek such essentials and having the cognitive wherewithal to find or create more of them more efficiently (e.g., by making tools and eventually planting crops) gave hominins an advantage that many bigger and stronger creatures lacked. As the millennia went by, this exploring, learning, planning, and choosing branch of the primate family did very well at Darwin's grand game, with one of its descendent species, *Homo sapiens*, becoming a presence on all continents and arguably the planet's dominant creature. There was however a liability within the species' mental apparatus: vulnerability to many disorders, including addiction.

Plant-based drugs have coexisted with *Homo sapiens* for thousands of years and probably tens of thousands of years. Fruit that became overripe would ferment, and tobacco, the coca plant, cannabis, the areca nut, and the opium poppy grew wild in some parts of the world. Some human beings sampled them as they did other consumables in the environment.

What was unique about some of the substances within these plants is that they were highly reinforcing even though they were not nutritive. Ingesting opium could be a more positive experience than drinking water even though humans do not need opium to survive but will die without water. Drinking alcohol could become more rewarding than having sex or cuddling a newborn, even though natural selection has made the latter two experiences intensely pleasurable because members of the species who found them aversive would have had less chance of passing on their genes.

The remarkable decision making system of our species has a design flaw, namely overvaluing from an evolutionary perspective the particular class of consumables we call addictive drugs. The human brain functions via an extraordinarily complex system of neurotransmitters, receptors, and circuits that helps humans make critical survival decisions such as recognizing and orienting ourselves to important stimuli and learning and remembering associations between environmental features (e.g., food), our behavior (e.g., eating), and consequences for ourselves and for others (e.g., we like the taste or we don't).

Neurotransmitters such as dopamine and serotonin have particular shapes that allow them to bind to specific receptors on brain cells (neurons) much as certain keys will fit in certain locks. This binding can activate, suppress, or modulate the strength and nature of a signal between different neurons and brain regions.

All addictive drugs have natural parallels within the human brain that bind to receptors that evolved to respond to endogenous chemicals. For instance, heroin binds to the same receptors as the endorphins and enkephalins that the human body produces naturally. This allows addictive drugs to trigger neural effects that evolved for other purposes. Perhaps the most important of these for addiction is the release of the neurotransmitter dopamine. Dopamine release is by no means the only process involved in helping an organism learn that a particular behavior or stimulus is highly rewarding, but it is centrally involved. To put it colloquially, dopamine release is how the brain tells you, "The behavior you just did was good for you and you should expect it will benefit you again the next time."

Brain imaging studies show that most addictive drugs cause a spike in release of dopamine far exceeding that of rewards that are more important for survival. Subjectively, even users who have had many naturally rewarding experiences in their lives may find that use of a drug exceeds those rewards. And behavioral observation confirms that people will devote far more time and energy to obtaining addictive drugs than they will many other rewards in the environment, even if those natural rewards are central to survival.

Like all other forms of learning, with repetition of the consumptive behavior, the association of the drug with its effect and the anticipation that the next use will also be rewarding become stronger. But with addictive drug use, the anticipation of future reward does not track reality as well as it does for other behaviors. In addiction, even as tolerance sets in and reduces reward from drug use, and harms accrue increasing the punishing effects of drug use, the human brain still anticipates that future drug use will be extremely rewarding. Subjectively, this creates the experience of not liking drug use as much as before but wanting it just as much, because the reward anticipation function within the brain has been corrupted. This corrupted learning process can become deeply entrenched even as the damage of drug use escalates, up to and including potentially fatal consequences.

At least some portion of our species have had, depending on where they lived, access to at least some plant-based drugs for millennia. Most cultures developed norms and rituals constraining where and when and by whom drugs could be consumed, which likely limited the proportion of exposed individuals who became addicted. These are however imperfect controls on human behavior and thus we can be sure that addiction is a syndrome that has existed in at least some small proportion of our species since before written history. But comparing that truism to the human population's addiction problem in the past 150 years is like comparing a puddle formed by rainwater with the Atlantic Ocean. So what happened?

Something new: modern technology, biochemistry, and commerce

The preceding section may make it sound as if addiction is "just another brain disease" but that would be a misunderstanding. Yes, our brains evolved in a way that makes particular molecules very appealing to us, to the point that we will harm ourselves to obtain and consume them. But brains always exist in an environment with which we interact through our behavior, and if not for some dramatic changes in those variables, addiction would have remained a minor problem for our species rather than the massive public health and safety challenge it has become.

Although countless factors can contribute to addiction, as mentioned only one is truly necessary for it: consumption of available addictive drugs. Understanding how the availability and nature of such drugs has changed throughout human history is critical for appreciating why addiction is such a prevalent problem today. The brains of *Homo sapiens* today are essentially the same the species possessed two centuries ago, but the world in which those brains exist is utterly different.

A thinking, planning species that is highly attuned to taking drugs will eventually figure out how to make drugs and how to take them in more efficient ways. Consider some technological developments along these lines which happened in a very narrow window of time from the perspective of the tens of thousands of years of human evolution (see Box: Technological developments in drugs, drug taking, and drug accessibility in the past 175 years).

The developments are of different kinds. Some were in mechanical engineering. The hollow steel hypodermic needle allowed the injection of any drug that could take liquid form. This produces an extremely potent reinforcing effect—swallowing an opioid pill creates a slower onset, lower intensity response in the brain than does melting that pill and injecting the liquid directly into a vein. Cigarette rolling machines were another key mechanical innovation. Cigarettes used to be hand-rolled, and a skilled worker could produce perhaps one per minute. The first rolling machines increased the efficiency of this process 60-fold, and the modern descendants of those machines increased it 20,000-fold. This allowed cheap mass production, which translated into more population exposure.

Other innovations came from either extracting drugs from processed plant matter (e.g., heroin) or synthesizing them in a laboratory (e.g., amphetamine). Such drugs were purer and more potent than those found in nature, and could be efficiently mass produced.

The nature of other drugs was changed to make them more attractive. The wild tobacco plant is hard to inhale when smoked, and there were only a dozen documented cases of tobacco-induced lung cancer worldwide prior to 1900. But with the arrival of modern tobacco companies with technical knowhow, tobacco was blended to be sweeter and easier to inhale deeply, thus making smoking both more addictive and more likely to cause lung cancer.

The cigarette industry, which marketed and sold the most profitable product of the 20th century, is also the best example of a new environmental feature of modern addiction: mass

Technological developments in drugs, drug taking, and drug accessibility in the past 175 years

1853 Hollow steel hypodermic needle invented

1859 Cocaine synthesized

1864 Barbiturates synthesized

1867 Cigarette rolling machine invented

1874 Heroin synthesized

1887 Amphetamines synthesized

1893 Methamphetamine synthesized

1913 Blended tobacco cigarettes introduced

1949 Commercial jet age begins

1955 Benzodiazepines synthesized

1969 ARPAnet, an Internet precursor, is created

1991 World Wide Web invented

marketing. The industry was remarkably adept at changing norms in a pro-smoking direction. For example, because cigarette smoking was seen as feminine, the industry supplied cigarettes to soldiers during World War I and then circulated photos of grizzled, brave men in combat puffing away, fueling an explosion of smoking on the home front.

Other technologies helped globalize tobacco addiction. In the age of jet travel and the Internet, rather than only being able to use tobacco if it happened to grow nearby or was within the ambit of a delivery truck, essentially everyone on earth has access to tobacco. That's why today more people die of tobacco-induced lung cancer every 10 seconds than died of it through all of human history until the 20th century. The alcohol industry and the pharmaceutical industry both became global powerhouses, marketing their products in virtually every country and thereby exposing more people to addictive drugs.

Global commerce also creates huge incentives for multinational corporations to spread addiction. Consumption of addictive drugs is highly skewed such that the top 10 percent of consumers may consume as much as the rest of the population. In a capitalist economy, an addicted person is the best of all customers, so the incentives of companies (or of illicit drug trafficking organizations) is to generate as much addiction as possible. Setting aside morals, the objective reality is that corporations are very successful at this endeavor throughout the world.

The addictive drug-saturated environment in which our species exists today has grown up in less than two centuries. Because this is an eye-blink from the perspective of human evolution, the brains of *Homo sapiens* are essentially the same as they were when it all started. This is why it is overly simplistic to say that addiction is a brain disease without considering the context in which our brains exist. It would make more sense to say that addiction is a problem (or disease or disorder) that became prevalent when our long-evolved brain encountered a drug-rich environment and began to engage with it and indeed add further drugs to it through our combined powers and liabilities.

Just as a species that evolved to pursue calories when they were scarce becomes afflicted with an epidemic of obesity when more than enough calories are readily available, our species has an epidemic of addiction in response to the almost unimaginable increase in the availability and variety of potent drugs in recent centuries. This change in our environment is why at a population level the human species is experiencing so much more addiction now than for most of our evolutionary history. But let's ask a different question: Why isn't everyone addicted, given the unprecedented access to drugs? Or to put it another way, what changes the risk of addiction in the presence of an abundance of drugs?

Risk and protective factors for addiction

Risk factors and protective factors are sometimes discussed separately, but are really two sides of the same coin, for example, having parents who are addicted to alcohol is a risk factor for developing alcohol addiction and having parents without alcohol addiction is a protective factor against developing alcohol addiction. These factors can exist in individuals (e.g., genes), in environments (e.g., availability of drugs), and in the transaction between the two. Some of the factors discussed below are present at several of these levels at once, for example religious faith is an individual level variable but also an environmental one because one's family's and community's religious beliefs and practices will affect the individual too. All the factors below can affect the likelihood of addiction in a population or an individual in two ways, namely changing the likelihood that drugs are used at all and changing the likelihood that drug use will progress to addiction.

Availability. Because you cannot become addicted to a drug you don't use, by definition addiction risk is lower if a drug isn't available and hence can't be used. Global commerce has made some drugs, most notably alcohol and tobacco, available to an unprecedented degree, but even they vary in availability and drugs that aren't legally sold by world-spanning industries even more so.

Availability is rarely an on/off switch and more a matter of degree. Age-based purchasing laws for tobacco and alcohol can sometimes be evaded by youth, for example with a fake identification card or an amenable older sibling or friend. That said, they reduce the relative access of youth to alcohol and tobacco, thereby reducing their rates of problematic substance use. Government-operated

unprecedented access to drugs? Or to put it another way, what changes the risk of addiction in the presence of an abundance of drugs?

Risk and protective factors for addiction

Risk factors and protective factors are sometimes discussed separately, but are really two sides of the same coin, for example, having parents who are addicted to alcohol is a risk factor for developing alcohol addiction and having parents without alcohol addiction is a protective factor against developing alcohol addiction. These factors can exist in individuals (e.g., genes), in environments (e.g., availability of drugs), and in the transaction between the two. Some of the factors discussed below are present at several of these levels at once, for example religious faith is an individual level variable but also an environmental one because one's family's and community's religious beliefs and practices will affect the individual too. All the factors below can affect the likelihood of addiction in a population or an individual in two ways, namely changing the likelihood that drugs are used at all and changing the likelihood that drug use will progress to addiction.

Availability. Because you cannot become addicted to a drug you don't use, by definition addiction risk is lower if a drug isn't available and hence can't be used. Global commerce has made some drugs, most notably alcohol and tobacco, available to an unprecedented degree, but even they vary in availability and drugs that aren't legally sold by world-spanning industries even more so.

Availability is rarely an on/off switch and more a matter of degree. Age-based purchasing laws for tobacco and alcohol can sometimes be evaded by youth, for example with a fake identification card or an amenable older sibling or friend. That said, they reduce the relative access of youth to alcohol and tobacco, thereby reducing their rates of problematic substance use. Government-operated retail alcohol outlets such as exist in Sweden and in some US states also reduce access to alcohol by restricting sales to designated times and sites (and also, not incidentally, being better than private outlets at verifying purchaser age). Regions with government-run retail monopolies have lower rates of alcohol-related problems (e.g., impaired driving and fatalities, youth binge drinking) than regions with privatized sales outlets. Even in places with an entirely privatized liquor sale system, areas with lower density of outlets have fewer alcohol-related problems.

Prohibiting manufacture and sale of certain drugs is also a matter of degree. There are black markets in cocaine, heroin, and other illegal drugs. But prohibition does dramatically reduce the availability of those drugs, which is a key reason why addiction to even a single legal drug (tobacco) is more common than addiction to all illegal drugs combined.

When availability of a drug increases, addiction to that drug becomes more common. The explosion of cheap, strong gin in early 18th-century England led to a sixfold increase in consumption and a dramatic increase in alcohol-related morbidity and mortality. Beginning in the mid-1990s, opioid manufacturers in the US and Canada successfully pushed doctors to dramatically increase opioid prescribing. This pushed the per capita volume of prescribed opioids up 400 percent in a little more than a decade, triggering the deadly addiction and overdose crisis with which both of those nations are still grappling (Figure 2).

Rising prices can make a drug less available even if it physically exists at the same level. The most obvious example of this is when a drug is subjected to a tax—the day after the tax goes into effect, there are just as many cigarettes in the stores, but they are less accessible because fewer people can afford them. The Gin Craze of early 18th-century England was brought under control by parliamentary-imposed taxes on the drink and those who sold it.

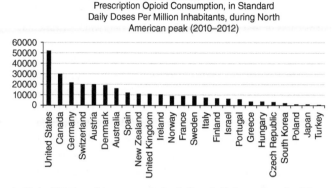

International Comparision of
Prescription Opioid Consumption, in Standard
Daily Doses Per Million Inhabitants, during North
American peak (2010–2012)

2. United Nations data on per capita daily opioid doses show the US and Canada became extreme outliers.

As a person's time is effectively part of the cost of a drug, increasing "search times" also can be thought of as a raise in price and a decline in availability, with alcohol state stores being one example and law enforcement closing down an open air drug market being another. In the other direction, Internet-based drug markets offering home delivery increase availability even at the same financial price, and therefore likely increase drug use and addiction.

Values and norms. Even when drugs are widely available, a significant proportion of the population chooses not to use drugs, which reduces their risk of addiction to zero no matter how many other risk factors they may carry. At the other end of the continuum are people who choose to use available drugs with great enthusiasm. A key factor shaping such decisions is the values and norms to which people are exposed and which they have internalized.

Imagine for example a Londoner growing up in an Iraqi immigrant community on Edgware Road. That individual will likely absorb the community values that cast drug use and intoxication as morally wrong. Even if they have doubts about the correctness of that view in their own mind, they will be aware that their family and community values are reflected in norms of behavior, for example they may be shunned by others if they engage in drug use. In contrast, imagine a Londoner growing up in Shoreditch in a bohemian family in which drug use is seen as a sign of liberation and self-exploration, and with a network of friends who see drug use in a similarly positive light. Relative to the bohemian, the Edgware Road dweller is more likely to think drug use is wrong and more likely to worry about negative social reactions if they use drugs. For both reasons they will be less likely to use drugs at all and to develop a drug problem.

Globally, the most prevalent factor shaping human beings' values and norms is religion. Most religions inveigh against substance use, intoxication, or both. Like all religious prohibitions, these are imperfectly followed, but are still robust predictors at the group level. Indeed, if you could ask one question to predict whether a US newborn will avoid becoming a drug using teenager, the smartest question to ask would not address their race, class, genes, or parent's substance use. Instead, you should ask whether the child will be raised in a religiously observant home, which is the best predictor of avoiding substance use problems (with Judaism, Mormonism, and Islam being the most protective).

In addition to blanket proscriptions against some drugs and some patterns of drug use (e.g., chronic drunkenness), religions sometimes endorse drug use in a specific, sacred context. Multiple religions encourage consumption of hallucinogenic drugs in particular ceremonies. Some Christian denominations serve wine at communion. It may seem odd that allowing use could discourage use, but consider the larger implicit message: If taking peyote is something done in a special context at a special time, then it is something not done outside of that special context and time (which covers 99.9 percent of existence).

Cultural forces also shape values and norms around drug use. Sometimes these cultural forces were or are religious in origin, sometimes not. Cultural values for example can be shaped by corporate activity. Mass media advertising portraying drug use as positive, exciting, sexy, fun, and free of risk will eventually be reflected in the values and norms of the culture, as the experience of the tobacco and alcohol industry has proven again and again (Figures 3 and 4). Cultural views about gender roles are also powerful shapers of behavior: societies in which women's substance use is frowned on have much larger differences between male and female rates of addiction than do cultures in which women's substance use is accepted or even lionized as a sign of liberation.

Cultures also vary in how much they value individualistic pleasure and autonomy relative to family and communal interests. Wealthier societies are more individualistic, with the US being a leading example. In such cultures, the idea of, for example, spending the evening at the bar when your children are at home, may be seen as more acceptable than it would in a society that presumed that individual satisfaction should always take a back seat to family and community needs.

Family values and norms also influence the likelihood of drug use and addiction. This occurs through the normal developmental forces, that is, in the same way that families influence members' values in all areas. It can also occur through an indirect route, namely that families that believe drug use is acceptable are more likely to have them available in the home. Teenaged experimentation with alcohol is facilitated when parents have a generously stocked liquor cabinet.

Family norms also shape whether youthful drug use increases or decreases over time, with consequent impact on the long-term risk for addiction. Some families would react to an adolescent smoking cannabis negatively, perhaps by imposing some restrictions on their child's activities in response. In other families, the same use would

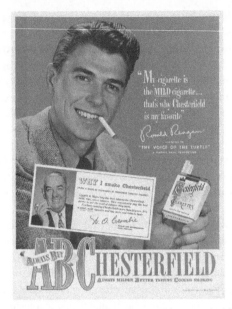

Addiction

3. Movie actor and future US President Ronald Reagan hawks Chesterfield cigarettes.

be viewed as a natural part of growing up and worthy of no comment, or perhaps even meet with some sign of approval. Families with drug use supportive norms are more likely to raise children who use drugs and whose drug use progresses to addiction.

Like all other risk and protective factors for addiction other than drug use per se, norms and values have a probabilistic impact. There are individuals whose own substance use behavior is the opposite of what would generally be predicted by the norms and values at play in their culture, community, and family. These can be broken down into "forbidden fruit" and "repulsion" effects.

Forbidden fruit effects refer to the fact that a subset of people want to use drugs precisely because they are widely considered

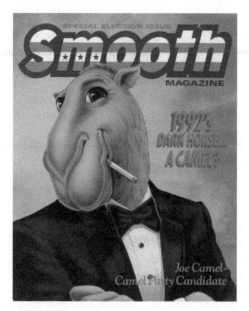

4. The Joe Camel tobacco logo was abandoned when advocates argued
it targeted children.

wrong or dangerous or unhealthy by people around them. This
could be an individual with an antisocial nature, in which case
they would also be more likely to engage in other antisocial
behaviors such as lying, stealing, destroying property, or worse.
But rebellion against social norms can also take more mundane
forms, for example some adolescents using drugs because they
want to demonstrate independence from authority and also be
witnessed by their peers defying parents, teachers, and other
adults who tell them what to do.

Repulsion effects operate in the other direction. Some people who
grow up in heavy drinking families and communities are so put off
by it that they never touch a drop. Across a society with a
historically serious alcohol problem, this may help explain why

entire generations of young people choose to drink much less than their elders, as is the case in England currently. There are also adolescents who react to current peer pressure to use drugs by making a point of never doing so.

Forbidden fruit effects and repulsion effects are potent for some individuals. But at the population level, they are small compared to the impact of values and norms in shaping drug use decisions and behaviors consistent with what is considered right and wrong, acceptable and unacceptable.

Environmental stressors and rewards. In Bruce Alexander's famous "Rat Park" experiment, conducted in Vancouver in the 1970s, rats that had a chance to interact and to engage in other diverting behaviors (e.g., running in the wheel) were less likely to become addicted to an available solution containing an opioid than rats kept alone in cages. Although the implications of this study have been wildly overstated (e.g., some people concluded drugs aren't really addictive in themselves, but the Rat Park effect didn't replicate with non-opioids or across species of rats either), the demonstration is important to understanding addiction in animals and may have relevance for human use of drugs as well.

Humans evolved to seek rewards and to choose among the rewards in our environment. Assuming a person has started to use drugs and experienced that reward, their likelihood of continuing to use them will probably be shaped by whether they have competing rewards available to them (e.g., a good job, a loving family, fun things to do) or their life is more like that of a caged rat. As the Beat writer William Burroughs put it, "You become a narcotics addict because you do not have strong motivations in the other direction. Junk wins by default." This effect is not universal—plenty of people with reward-filled lives become addicted—but it should nonetheless not be dismissed.

Stressful environments may raise the risk of addiction among those who use drugs, by increasing the negative reinforcement value of use (i.e., the short-term relief from fear, anxiety, depression). Stress can come in many forms including community or family disorder, exposure to violence (either as a victim or as a bystander), and racial and ethnic persecution.

Some believe that drug use and addiction are merely symptoms of poverty and economic inequality in a society. The research on this proposition is generally unsupportive. In Europe, alcohol problems among the young are higher rather than lower in more economically egalitarian societies. Australian surveys show that among lower income people, attaining increased economic security (e.g., getting a job, having one's income rise) predicts increased consumption of tobacco and alcohol. Globally, when societies begin to develop and become wealthier, their consumption of addictive drugs soars. Further, within societies, the highest rates of abstention tend to be among the poorest groups. So although there are many good reasons to attempt to reduce poverty, promising that this will reduce drug use and addiction is unwise.

Genes and personality traits. Many people have observed that addiction runs in families. Although part of this is due to shared environment, even children raised apart from an addicted parent are more likely to develop an addiction themselves. The effect is not consistent in size across drugs or sexes, but is real.

This does not mean however, as is sometimes stated in the popular press, that there is such a thing as being "born addicted." Even if an addicted mother has been using drugs during pregnancy, the newborn would have no learned association between drug use behavior and drug reinforcement, and hence its brain would not be altered in that fashion even if the mother's drug use caused other forms of damage.

To carry genes that put one at risk for addiction is not destiny, because again, if someone does not use a drug, they will not become addicted to it. Genes can increase risk by increasing the odds that one will seek drugs, but their more powerful contribution is to influence the effects that drugs have once taken.

Genes can shape propensity for becoming addicted to the drugs a person takes in two broad addiction-specific ways. One is through drug liking, that is, the drug simply feels better or worse for the user than for most other people, even before having any learning history with it. An example is the gene common in Han Chinese which inhibits the enzyme that breaks down alcohol, producing an unpleasant "Asian flush" response that discourages most people with this genetic heritage from becoming regular drinkers. Other people with no drug use history find that even at first use a drug is even more enjoyable to them than to most people who use it. Being on the positive end of the human variation in subjective reaction to drugs clearly has a genetic component and makes continued use and addiction more likely.

Genes can also change negative consequences of drug use. For example, sons of alcohol-addicted fathers are more likely to be able to "drink their mates under the table." They acquire tolerance more quickly and they have less severe hangovers. These might seem desirable traits until one remembers that unpleasant experiences with alcohol are often a warning sign that one is drinking too much. By not having to endure the punishment that most heavy drinkers would, it's easier for men with this genetic load to continue to drink heavily, thereby increasing their likelihood of becoming addicted to alcohol.

Genes can also affect risk of addiction through a non-specific pathway, namely by transmitting personality traits that are relevant to many domains of behavior, including but not limited to drug use. This should not be confused with the claim that there is such a thing as an "addictive personality." The hypothesis is usually never specified in enough detail to test it, but for what it's worth addicted people cover the full range of every dimension of human personality. Some are uptight and traditional; some are laid back and unconventional; some are angry and domineering; others are sad and reserved.

In contrast, particular individual personality traits influenced by genetics can matter. The most obvious candidates are sensation seeking and impulsivity. The former is the tendency to be drawn to novel stimuli in the environment. The latter is the tendency to have low self-control, for example, tending to leap before you look. Both traits are overrepresented among people who develop drug addiction, and it is easy to imagine causal pathways that could explain why this is more than a chance correlation.

Sex and age. Being young or male, or even more, being a young male, is a robust predictor of being more likely to use addictive drugs in virtually every culture throughout the world. There are many non-competing reasons for this, including greater willingness to and social acceptability to explore and break with conventions, social forces (e.g., what one's peer group is doing), role socialization (e.g., to drink is manly, to be young is to go to parties), as well as freedom granted from other responsibilities (e.g., child care) that would compete with use. Widespread negative attitudes and associations regarding women's substance use (e.g., with immorality) also help account for the difference. Biological factors are also likely at play in that the same amount of drug use may extract more toll on the old than the young, and females than males, reducing willingness to continue to engage in the behavior.

In particular cultural moments, there are exceptions to these heuristics. In an effort to stimulate business, the alcohol industry launched advertising campaigns to portray drinking as positive to women, which was effective at bringing women's alcohol consumption closer to males in the US in recent decades. In the

US and Europe, the current generation of young people is rather abstemious for reasons that are much debated (e.g., whether it has to do with the greater appeal of the Internet), meaning that in multiple countries their rate of substance use and addiction is far less than what is seen in the Baby Boomer generation.

Mental health. The co-occurrence of addiction and psychiatric disorders is very high. Although it has been argued at times that the pairings of mental illness and drugs are specific (e.g., anxious people become addicted to drugs with anxiolytic effects, depressed people to drugs with stimulant effects), the association seems to be generic. For example, people with schizophrenia have higher rates of tobacco, alcohol, cannabis, and stimulant addiction—drugs with different pharmacological effects—than people with good mental health. There are many theories as to why the positive association between worse mental health and addiction comes about.

Many specialists and non-specialists explain the co-occurrence by interpreting addictive substance use by people with mental illness as "self-medication," which is an unfortunate term for several reasons. First, addictive drug use is not medicinal in that virtually every study conducted has found that the course of psychiatric disorders is more severe and destructive when an individual has a co-occurring addiction. Second, the explanation is unintentionally dehumanizing in that it denies the possibility that a person with mental illness might use drugs for the same reasons any other person would (e.g., just because you are depressed doesn't mean raising a champagne toast at your child's wedding has anything to do with your depression).

Three other explanations for the high comorbidity of addiction and psychiatric disorder seem more plausible. First, many psychiatric problems limit the ability of people to complete complex tasks requiring extensive planning, self-control, and attention. Recovery from addiction is one such task, such that if two people who smoke in precisely the same way attempt the challenging task of quitting, the one who is depressed is less likely to succeed just as they would be less likely to succeed if the two were trying to lose 10 pounds or successfully manage their diabetes. Second, negative reinforcement may be a more prominent effect of drugs in people with psychiatric disorder, that is, if one is consumed with depression, anxiety, traumatic memories, or frightening hallucinations the oblivion some drugs offer may be more appealing than if one generally experiences psychological well-being.

The third explanation for the co-occurrence is of a different sort. As mentioned, we characterize addiction as a syndrome we believe links a bunch of observable indicators such as tolerance, withdrawal, harm, craving, and the like. Psychiatric disorders are also generally inferred rather than directly observed: there is no blood test for depression, no X-ray for bipolar disorder, and no neuroimaging signature for post-traumatic stress disorder. Because all the boundaries between psychiatric disorders are best guesses at how to carve nature at its joints, some of the boundaries are likely drawn incorrectly. In other words, a particular deficit or liability in the brain might express itself as addiction in one person, as depression in another, and as both in a third person. The "co-occurrence" of psychiatric and addictive disorders could thus sometimes be a diagnostic mistake made by calling a single disorder two distinct disorders.

The other side of the coin is that good mental health appears to lower the risk of becoming addicted. Good mental health includes capacities such as the ability to recognize and manage one's emotions, to cope successfully with stress, and to complete difficult tasks. All of these capacities reduce the likelihood that drug use will progress to addiction and probably also make it more likely that an addicted person is able to enter recovery.

Social networks. Drug use—like virtually all other human behavior—is shaped by the people around us. Having a social network in which drug use is prevalent and accepted increases the likelihood that a person will initiate, continue, or return to use drugs, and having a social network with little or no drug use will exert the opposite impact. This comes about both through practical realities (i.e., drugs are more or less available) as well as through the desire for shared experiences within social networks, and the effects of social approval or disapproval on behavior.

Studies with young children show that even before drug use has entered the life of a cohort, social network effects are important. Children who bond with pro-social peers are less likely to go on to develop drug problems than are those who bond with antisocial peers or with no peers at all.

Social network effects are sometimes dismissed on the basis that people choose their social networks and therefore any association between say higher rates of drug use in a social network and by individuals within it merely reflects people choosing to associate with those with similar interests and values. This is empirically wrong in the case of children and adolescents, whose social networks are heavily shaped by forces beyond their control, that is, their elders and also by the state (e.g., legal compulsion to attend school puts one in touch with a particular social network). Adults have more freedom to pick social networks, but even this is limited: One cannot choose to whom one is related by blood, who lives next door, or whom one's employer hires. And even when one can choose (e.g., whom to marry), there is no contradiction between assuming that individuals choose social networks and are then affected by those networks, for example a college student may choose to associate with other students who seem "edgy" and exciting, and once in such circles have opportunities to use drugs that they did not expect.

Chapter 4
Recovery and treatment

Despite addiction's life-destroying potential and fierce hold on those who experience it, recovery is not unusual. Millions of people around the world participate in peer-led mutual help fellowships that assist them to stop their destructive substance use, repair damaged relationships, improve their health and well-being, and succeed in role obligations. Millions of others walk the same path by accessing some form of professionally provided treatment. And even larger numbers recover without any specialty assistance at all. In recovery, much of what was lost in addiction is regained, and some recovering people maintain that their lives are richer and their functioning better after recovery than it was before their addiction began.

The term "recovery from addiction" is used in different ways in different contexts. For one person addicted to heroin, this may involve lifetime use of a substitution medication such as buprenorphine whereas for another it involves lifetime commitment to the "12-step" mutual help organization Narcotics Anonymous. For one person addicted to alcohol it could involve lifetime abstinence, for another it could involve a period of abstinence transitioning back to occasional but non-destructive social drinking.

Within 12-step mutual help organizations and the many professionally operated treatment programs they have influenced, recovery refers to lifetime abstinence from drugs coupled with greater compassion for and service to others, restitution to those one has harmed, and a spiritual state of serenity. People who define recovery in this way tend to think of it as a core part of their personal identity. Particularly in the early years, recovery becomes a central life goal and preoccupation, with many experiences and relationships being interpreted through that lens. For the rest of their lives, even after years or decades of recovery, such people tend to identify as and may also describe themselves as "a person in long-term recovery."

Because recovery typically involves significant work to attain and maintain, it often brings increased feelings of worth to the individual, particularly in contrast to the years of active addiction. This is often reflected in others' eyes as well, in that people in recovery are generally respected more than people who display signs of serious addiction.

In recovery from addiction, many people experience improvement in the central relationships of their lives (see Box: How recovery from addiction improves relationships). The box features the prototypic experience of recovery and one that many people will know because it has been portrayed in many movies, television shows, and biographies. But survey research shows that many people who resolve a serious addiction tread a less dramatic path. They do not use the term "recovery" nor do they see their addiction history as central to who they are. For them, it was "a difficult period," "a misspent youth," "a self-destructive phase," and the like, without any important connection to their current life situation or sense of identity. Some of these individuals may abstain forever from drugs, but others may continue using at a lower level that does less harm to themselves and others.

How recovery from addiction improves relationships—one woman's story

The American recovery advocate Ryan Hampton has collected many stories of addiction and recovery posted with consent on-line. This is an excerpt from one of those stories, told by Hannah:

> My daughter began to stay with me, she began to trust that I wasn't going away again. I was on my own journey of forgiving myself for what I had put her through, how I hadn't been there. I had missed her so much, and every moment with her was gold. I was given the gift of that sight.
>
> My family began to forgive me. I had hurt everyone and there was a lot of anger to work through. They loved me through all of this, and I had to learn to be okay with them feeling however they felt.
>
> My relationship with my partner grew. We learned we could love each other without drugs. Seriously, that was tough. I didn't know if we were going to make it, and I had gotten to a point where I was okay with that. Part of me thinks our relationship survived because I was willing to let it go for my sobriety.

Severity of addiction is a significant predictor of how someone pursues and defines recovery. In a sample of people with serious alcohol problems, improving groups tend to split into a pathway of people who become permanently abstinent and those who return to moderate drinking. The former group usually starts their journey with greater physical dependence on alcohol (e.g., blackouts, withdrawal), higher levels of consumption, and lower social capital (e.g., high rates of divorce and employment) than does the latter group and over time is more likely to access AA and professional addiction treatment. At least some of the latter group would not meet the criteria for addiction even though they engaged in harmful drinking, and the care seeking of this group might be more along the lines of brief consultation with a physician or psychotherapist, or, no outside help at all.

If an addiction has destroyed your health and your life, your recovery is more likely to become central to your life story and identity than it would if you had a low severity addiction that did not upend your existence. Likewise, if you have not built up high physical dependence on a drug, it is easier to return to using it moderately (including after a period of abstinence) than if you are physically dependent on it. Finally, your recovery pathway will be influenced by those to whom you come into contact, such that a heavily addicted person may find an AA meeting comfortable and that the AA story of alcohol addiction and recovery fits their experience, whereas a less addicted person may find that AA members seem much worse off and difficult to relate to, and fit in better in a mutual help group like Moderation Management, which helps problem drinking individuals return to less harmful alcohol consumption.

How people think about recovery and pursue it is in some ways a creative, subjective process of defining identity and forming a life narrative. But it also has the objective component of severity of addiction influencing the process, for example, someone whose life has in fact been destroyed by a drug and who is severely addicted to it is going to have a very hard time returning to moderate use and convincing themselves and other people that their addiction was "just a phase."

Rates of and pathways to recovery

For some disorders, for example cancers, scientists have excellent information on people's odds of recovery over various time intervals. The addiction field possesses relatively less precise information, but some important data points are available.

The first is that recovery often requires multiple efforts. Across addictions, most people who succeed in abstaining from a drug have tried to do so before, often multiple times. Relapse is common across every addiction discussed in this book, even after periods of abstinence. This demonstrates how well ingrained addictive substance use becomes in the brain, in learned behavior, and in life contexts. In recovery, addicted people must maintain a level of vigilance over a longer period and across a broader range of situations than they would if they had recovered from an acute health problem, such as a torn Achilles tendon, a bout of influenza, or a fractured bone.

The second finding is that recovery even from quite serious addictions is possible. Although his sample was all white, male, and American, it's useful to know that the Harvard University psychiatrist George Vaillant found that about half of adults diagnosed with what was then called "alcoholism" eventually recovered. Encouragingly, of those who abstained from alcohol for four years, 90 percent abstained for the rest of their lives.

The third finding is that recovering from addiction is a common experience. National survey data show that over 9 percent of the US adult population (22.3 million people) describe themselves as having had a serious substance use problem in the past but not having one now.

Finally, the majority of recoveries happen among people who did not receive specialty addiction treatment. This is not as surprising as it may seem. Life happens, and addicted people will experience many things in life that are more enduring in their impact than any treatment they might seek.

A man who has tried and failed to quit smoking for years is overcome with love and a sense of responsibility upon seeing his newborn child for the first time; he stubs out his last smoke and never touches them again. A woman told by her doctor that she has the liver functioning of someone 30 years her senior may put down the bottle out of fear of an early grave. A cocaine using, disorganized, and depressed man may find that the structure, discipline, and sense of purpose to which he is exposed upon joining the military helps him walk away from drugs forever. And an opioid-addicted autoworker may give up his use when his company begins drug testing employees and announces that a positive test will result in termination of employment. Public policy changes may also stimulate efforts at recovery, for example a tobacco tax hike or a workplace smoking ban may tip the balance for some addicted smokers such that they quit.

Also, of course, there are many sources of support, advice, and alternative rewards beyond the addiction treatment system. The best known are mutual help organizations such as AA, but there are many others: parents, spouses, children, extended family, friends, co-workers, teachers, and faith community leaders are often important in helping people recover. In addition to support and information these individuals may also provide accountability and pressure (e.g., "I will end our relationship if you keep using cocaine") that spurs someone to seek recovery.

The mantra "There are many pathways to recovery" thus has a solid basis in fact. Any given recovering person may understandably feel that their own pathway is the best for everyone, but the best path for any given individual is whatever moves them from a point where their addiction is doing great harm to where they can live a healthier, more fulfilling, and meaningful life. Religions teach that there is only one way to get to heaven, but when it comes to addiction recovery, we should all just be grateful that someone has arrived by whichever route they travelled.

Addiction treatment

As mentioned, many people recover from addiction without ever seeking addiction treatment. But millions of other people access addiction treatment each year, either because they find they cannot recover without it or because they are under pressure of some sort from what are sometimes described as the "4 Ls": Liver, lover, livelihood, or the law. What they encounter in treatment varies across and within countries, but it is possible to sketch the general contours and give a sense of the content and effects of addiction treatment on patients.

We should begin by correcting the common misunderstanding that addiction treatment is the same as "detox." Detoxification literally means "removing the poisons," but in practice means safely withdrawing an intoxicated individual from the drugs they have been using. There are two circumstances in which this occurs. One is in emergencies where a person has consumed so much of a drug (or combination of drugs) that they are completely incapacitated or at serious risk of harm. The second is more planned, for example when someone who is addicted to alcohol is trying to stop drinking at the beginning of a treatment episode.

Most people who receive detoxification are addicted. As we have noted, addiction is almost always coupled with dependence, such that the absence of the substance can trigger withdrawal symptoms that are usually aversive and sometimes dangerous. In a medical detoxification program, withdrawal is monitored closely and medications are given to make the process safer and less uncomfortable. Individuals going through this experience may be given a medication to replace the effects of the drug, for example receiving buprenorphine when withdrawing from heroin or benzodiazepines when withdrawing from alcohol. Such services are typically provided under supervision in the medical unit of a health care facility, although sometimes the addicted individual can stay at home during the process, reporting in once or several times a day to their care provider.

Some unethical for-profit agencies portray detoxification as the end of addiction, for example by promoting rapid detoxification under anesthesia as a 24-hour miracle cure. But detoxification is no more a treatment for addiction than emergency defibrillation is a treatment for the heart disease that caused a sudden cardiac arrest. A person leaves detoxification with the same brain, body, and learned behaviors as they entered, meaning they are still addicted. Only the acute effect of the drug has been removed. For this reason, detoxification should be followed up immediately with treatment for the addiction.

Addiction treatment is provided in a range of contexts. Any health care professional with a general practice might offer advice about addiction to a patient, but specialty care is offered in settings which take the care of addiction as their primary purpose. Four settings predominate (see Box: Settings for specialty addiction treatment).

Addiction treatment is a bit like a cafeteria, in that many things are offered and patients may differ in what they find beneficial. Most programs offer some or all of the components below.

A substance-free environment. Addiction treatment offers a substance-free environment for patients. This is particularly important when the person lives or works in a substance-saturated context, for example if they live with their parents or a spouse who also are addicted, or if they are homeless and spend their days with a group of fellow addicted individuals on the street. Being away from cues to use drugs and easy access to them increases the chance of making progress in treatment. Obviously this is easier to achieve in inpatient and residential settings than in outpatient care.

When the individual leaves treatment, they will typically return to their former environment, and this will in some cases heighten the potential for relapse. But even a temporary break provides an opportunity for the individual to withdraw from substances, stabilize physically and psychologically, and learn

Settings for specialty addiction treatment

Inpatient care is offered mainly in hospitals. A few of these hospitals specialize in addiction but more commonly inpatient programs are a ward within a psychiatric or general hospital. Inpatient programs have physicians and nurses on staff. They are fully equipped to safely manage withdrawal and to provide diagnostic tests and medications for addiction and the medical and psychiatric disorders with which it commonly co-occurs. Inpatient programs also typically have social workers and psychologists who provide additional care such as case management and individual or group psychotherapy. Patients stay in inpatient care 24 hours a day, typically for a period of weeks. Inpatient care was extremely common in developed Western countries 40 years ago, but such care has contracted dramatically since because it was often shown to be more expensive without increased effectiveness over care in other settings.

Residential care also requires the patient to live temporarily on site, usually for weeks and sometimes for months. It is far less "medicalized" than inpatient care, and is typically provided in buildings that feel more like a motel or camping lodge. Usually some medically trained staff are available and some medical services provided, but at lower levels than inpatient care. Because the staff to patient ratio is lower and patients stay longer, it is usually possible in residential settings to cultivate communal norms among patients to support recovery, and this may be accentuated by the provision of counseling to small or large groups.

Intensive outpatient care is a setting in which individuals receive care for hours a day (in some cases as many as 8 or 12) but do not stay overnight. This setting goes under many names

(continued)

including partial hospitalization and day treatment. Other than patients sleeping at home or in a nearby hotel each night, intensive outpatient care is otherwise similar to residential care.

Traditional outpatient care is provided in clinics similar to those managing many other chronic diseases (e.g., diabetes). Care providers may be medical professionals but are more often social workers, psychologists, or counselors. Patients visit the clinic only on the subset of days they receive care and do so for shorter intervals than in intensive outpatient care (e.g., 1–2 visits a week of 60–90 minutes each). Patients may receive medications in outpatient care, and will almost always receive some form of counseling in individual or group sessions.

skills to help them cope with the stresses and temptations of their daily environment.

Information and education. Treatment programs provide information about addiction in a variety of ways, including as a part of counseling, in the form of lectures and interactive presentations, and in printed materials. Information alone is not likely to help arrest addiction, but can be quite useful. For example, understanding that addiction is a chronic disorder may help persuade the individual that extended treatment is necessary. Knowing about how to access services may help the individual address addiction-related problems and also seek treatment again if they relapse. Provision of information on overdose identification and rescue techniques to patients and their families may save lives in a similar situation.

Emotional support and role modeling. Trying to recover from addiction can be hard work, and most people find that support from others makes the load easier to lift. Many treatment programs are social in nature, meaning that patients encounter other patients, for example in group psychotherapy. Support can come in many forms, including acceptance of addiction without shame or rebuke, recognition of positive steps taken for recovery, encouragement to attempt change, and a sense of fellowship with others on the same journey.

Role models can matter in all types of human learning, certainly including recovery from addiction. Role modeling can occur when patients earlier in the recovery process learn from those who are farther down the road they wish to travel. In some treatment programs there are staff members who are themselves in recovery from addiction that patients admire and try to emulate. Sometimes such individuals are in recovery because it's essential to their job (e.g., peer support specialists), in other cases they are physicians, social workers, nurses, psychologists, or other professionals who happen to be in recovery. A role model gives a patient an opportunity to copy that person's strategies and behavior. Role models also can inspire hope and build motivation to change.

Teaching cognitive and behavioral skills. Many treatments use a range of methods to help the addicted person master new skills that will help them recover. Cognitive skills are useful for attaining recovery and also more generically for dealing with stress, relationships with others, and maintaining a healthy self-concept. Such skills include learning to be aware of and interrupt dysfunctional thoughts (e.g., viewing every challenge as a catastrophe) and learning how to think flexibly (e.g., not seeing complex situations and people in black and white terms). In addiction care, particular attention is often devoted to helping patients track lines of thinking that precede relapse, as well as helping them think about relapse productively (e.g., "I made a mistake from which I can learn" rather than "I screwed up again because I am worthless"). Cultivating a habit of patience, that is, pausing to think before making major decisions or taking consequential actions, is another cognitive skill that can be learned in treatment and is particularly helpful to impulsive patients.

Other skills are behavioral and include things such as learning how to listen actively, how to handle offers to purchase or use drugs, and how to manage unpleasant emotions. Other behavioral skills that might be taught in treatment relate to daily functioning, for example how to manage one's daily schedule and how to act in a job interview. This can include learning how to manage stress, how to recognize signs of risk for relapse, and how to communicate better with friends and family.

Treatment programs have multiple methods of improving cognitive and behavioral skills. One of the most common is cognitive-behavioral therapy delivered in an individual or group setting. Didactic lectures may also be used. Behavioral skills can be practiced during treatment, and some long-term residential settings establish systems to reward behaviors like showing up on time, being responsible, and being respectful to other residents. Communication skills training is a specific type of such practice, which is usually done in vivo, for example when a therapist works with a couple or family of the patient and helps them observe and improve how they communicate. Also as mentioned, cognitive and behavioral skill acquisition can also be facilitated by patient-to-patient interaction and attendant role modeling.

Motivational interviewing. Addiction often brings ambivalence about change, because the short-term reinforcement of continued drug use sometimes seems more important than the larger but more distant rewards of recovery. Motivational interviewing is a style of counseling that addresses ambivalence head on by explicitly acknowledging the things patients like about drug use rather than trying to argue them away. Relieved of the need to defend themselves about enjoying some aspects of drug use, patients often become more candid about admitting the costs of their use to themselves and others.

Motivational interviewing works with the patient's own agenda rather than focusing on the desires of others for change. The logic is that while pressure from employers, loved ones, and police may lead some people to change, they are more likely to do so if they see that doing so would benefit themselves. A key tactic for doing this in motivational interviewing is asking the patient to articulate what they care about the most (e.g., being a good parent, succeeding at school, their freedom, money in their pocket), and then ask whether their addictive drug use helps or interferes with those priorities.

Contingency management. Contingency management is the application of the behavioral principle that human beings are more likely to do things that bring positive reinforcement and less likely to do things that result in a negative consequence. This principle had been applied for decades in "token economies" involving patients with serious psychiatric disorders, such as schizophrenia. But its application to addiction was uncertain for many years. At one point it was argued by many scientists that addicted individuals had no control over the drug use, but the American psychologist Stephen Higgins showed that in fact the offer of a small monetary reward for abstinence from cocaine as verified by urine analysis led many patients to refrain from using cocaine for the designated period. This indicated that addicted individuals generally had enough self-control to change drug use behavior in response to transparent, certain, and prompt rewards. Higgins and other scholars expanded this principle to show that a broad range of behaviors responded to such small rewards, including showing up to treatment sessions, filling out a job application, and going to 12-step mutual help group meetings.

Over 100 clinical trials have found favorable results from contingency management over a range of addictions. Contingency management can be used as a standalone treatment but more commonly is used to supplement other approaches.

Outside of voluntary treatment settings, contingency management also has proven effective in the criminal justice system. Such programs are generally known as "swift, certain, and fair" because rather than rely on harsh punishments, they focus on making consequences immediate and predictable (see Box: 24/7 Sobriety as a management strategy for people convicted of repeated alcohol-involved crimes).

24/7 Sobriety as a management strategy for people convicted of repeated alcohol-involved crimes

A county prosecutor named Larry Long became discouraged about seeing individuals with alcohol problems—some of whom he grew up with in South Dakota—cycle through court over and over for impaired driving convictions. Seizure of vehicles, suspension of driving licenses, and the threat of future imprisonment if intoxicated driving one day resulted in a fatality did not break the cycle. Long decided to allow these individuals to stay in the community and even to keep driving, instead using the power of the court to restrict their drinking.

Each morning and each evening enrollees in 24/7 Sobriety had to come in and blow into a breathalyzer to assess whether they have complied. If the test showed they had not been drinking, they were immediately rewarded with continued freedom. But if the test was positive, they were immediately arrested and given a very short jail sentence. Even though a single night in jail is not a long time for this population, most of whom have endured longer sentences in the past, the fact that this consequence is swift and certain is highly influential. Of the over 10 million breath tests that have been scheduled in South Dakota's program 99.1 percent have seen the individual complete the test and be shown to be abstinent. Not only did drunk driving arrests drop in the state, but so did domestic violence arrests and premature mortality. Other US States subsequently adopted the 24/7 Sobriety model.

The program also attracted attention in the United Kingdom, where it was piloted in London and found to be similarly successful at reducing alcohol consumption and related crime. It was then expanded across London and a few years later was rolled out nationwide. This was an important demonstration of the fact that basic behavioral principles concerning addictive drugs are not culturally bound.

Medications. Only a small number of medications are used in addiction treatment, far fewer, for example, than are used in the care of cancer or heart disease. Yet they have an important role, particularly in the care of people addicted to opioids and tobacco but also for those addicted to alcohol.

For some of the drugs to which people become addicted, there are medications that function as a stabilizing, lower intensity, less harmful replacement. For someone addicted to cigarettes, a nicotine patch may help them kick the habit of inhaling carcinogens without enduring nicotine withdrawal. For heroin and other opioids, the most widely employed replacement medication is called methadone. Methadone creates physical and psychological stability for about 24 hours per dose. This supplants the rollercoaster existence common in heroin addiction where an individual might go through cycles of intense drug reward followed soon by crashing withdrawal, followed by a desperate period of further drug seeking, one or more times per day.

Another sort of medication is designed to make the once-reinforcing experience of taking drugs neutral or even aversive. A drug known as disulfiram, for example, makes it hard for the body to break down alcohol, producing an unpleasant physical reaction in drinkers, including feeling sick to the stomach, that blood is rushing to the face, and the heart is pounding. A different medication, naltrexone, doesn't induce such unpleasant effects, but does reduce the positive feelings people get from consuming alcohol and opioids. The idea is that reduced pleasure from drug use, as well as knowledge by the user that pleasure will be less, will reduce drug use over time. Still other medications are intended to reduce craving. An example of such a medication is acamprosate, which is used to treat people addicted to alcohol.

Some people are puzzled or even upset at the use of medications for addiction, particularly substitute medications, remarking, "How can you treat drug addiction with drugs?", or more pointedly "How can you treat opioid addiction with another opioid?" An analogy might help: If someone accidentally cut themselves badly in the kitchen with a carving knife and the wound became infected to the point that surgery was required, a surgeon would likely use a scalpel (i.e., a knife) to open the wound so that it could be cleaned and then stitched. Yet we don't ask "How can you treat a knife wound with a knife?" because we know that there are different kinds of knives wielded by different people for different purposes. The same is true of medications for addiction. Yes, methadone is an opioid, but it is a different type of opioid than heroin, used by different people for a different purpose than is the person self-injecting heroin on the street.

Linkage to other resources, including mutual help groups. Many people who experience addiction have other significant medical, psychiatric, legal, housing, and employment problems. At one time it was believed that if the addiction were resolved, these other problems would evaporate, but this is not in fact the norm. Even problems directly initiated via addiction could take on an independent life of their own: a hepatitis C infection from sharing injection equipment doesn't vanish when the person stops injection drug use, the business that went bankrupt after an addiction led to poor decisions doesn't receive a new infusion of capital, the arrest for drunk driving is still on the record books. Quality addiction programs therefore nest themselves in a social service network to which they connect patients for aid during and after their contact with addiction treatment services.

Many addiction treatment programs also link patients to addiction-focused mutual help organizations. There are structured interventions that treatment programs can use to help individuals connect with these programs. These include "warm handoffs" in which patients are given an orientation to the nature of mutual help groups and introduced to an experienced member who will take them to a meeting. Another example is "12-step facilitation counseling," a therapy designed to provide direct benefit during care as well as connect the person to 12-step mutual help groups that will support their recovery after addiction treatment has ended.

Effectiveness of treatment

If we asked an oncologist whether cancer treatment really worked, we would immediately expect a bunch of clarifying questions: what treatment or combination of treatments? What type of cancer and at what site or sites in the body is it present? Was the cancer caught early or is it late stage? Is the patient organized, motivated, and well supported by a social network or will it be hard for them to follow a complex treatment regime? Yet, for whatever reason, many people expect the question of whether addiction treatment "works" or "how often it works" to be easily answerable.

Certainly addiction treatment has been extensively studied, including in what most scientists consider the "gold standard" design of a randomized clinical trial as well as in observational studies. All medications used in the field have been subjected to many clinical trials. Substitution drugs (e.g., methadone for heroin addiction, the nicotine patch for tobacco addiction) have generated strong evidence of benefit in such studies.

Medications like naltrexone that make substance use a neutral or negative experience generally "work" in the sense of producing the promised pharmacological and psychological effects, but they face a design problem: Once the person knows that they work, they may not be diligent about taking them every day. For this reason, the development of longer-acting medications is a significant breakthrough. This allows, for example, someone who is worried that their motivation to stop taking heroin will wane in a few days to essentially bind their own hands via a medication that lasts for a week or a month.

Medications simply aren't available for all addictions. Despite years of research and considerable financial investment, there is no effective medication for addiction to stimulants such as cocaine and methamphetamine. The only treatments for those addictions are psychosocial and behavioral, and thus treatment for these disorders may be less effective than that for other addictions.

Psychotherapies and behavioral therapies, whether provided in a residential setting or while a patient lives at home, can be very helpful. Good results have been found for treatments such as cognitive-behavioral psychotherapy, 12-step facilitation counseling, motivational enhancement counseling, and contingency management.

We can only talk very crudely about what the odds are that any given person will benefit from addiction treatment because people, addictions, and treatment vary so much. But judged at a glance the literature would suggest that 30–40 percent of people benefit a good deal. For some people that might mean they never use substances again, for others it will mean they cut back their use dramatically or have a long enough period of abstinence to secure some gains in their health and life situation. Perhaps another 20–30 percent benefit more modestly.

The remainder don't seem to benefit at all, at least from their current episode of care. Many of these people drop out of treatment very quickly. Others participate fully but do not change their behavior in any way. A sadly common situation is to see someone do very well in a four-week residential rehabilitation treatment program and relapse within a week of leaving—or even on the same day. This underscores the enduring nature of addiction and the need for long-term care and support. Multiple "rounds" of addiction treatment prior to recovery are common.

In the context of other chronic disorders with biological and behavioral components, such as diabetes, the effectiveness of addiction treatment looks much more positive. Conditions that can't be quickly cured by medication or surgery and require long-term change in many behaviors are simply challenging to treat. The proportion of times that addiction treatments work very well or partially is more impressive from that perspective.

Finally, one has to be humble in assessing whether a treatment has worked because the complexity of an individual's addiction doesn't always allow for simple answers. As mentioned, a grand "treatment success" may be revealed as a "four-week wonder" the day after they leave treatment and return to their drug use as if nothing had happened. In other cases a "failed treatment" episode plants a seed in an addicted person's life that takes years to flower. Many an AA meeting features a speaker who thanks the person who told them 20 years ago that they had a drinking problem and an apology to them "wherever they are" for telling them to go to hell.

The fact that many people benefit from treatment raises the question of why many addicted individuals don't want to seek treatment, or do so only because they are being pressured by a loved one, an employer, a health crisis, or the legal system. Recall the ambivalence that is common in addiction: With hard work over a long period, greater rewards are possible, but in the short term drugs continue to be highly reinforcing. Further, many of the biggest costs of addiction are inflicted on other people, and the addicted individual may therefore be less aware of or concerned about them than they would be about damage they experienced directly themselves. Indeed, recognition that some addicted people will choose to continue using drugs has led to the development of services focused on making the consequences of that use less dangerous, as described below.

Services focused on the consequences of drug use

Over the past 40 years, public health systems in many countries have diversified in their offerings of services to people who are addicted to drugs. Services focused on reducing or eliminating drug use and promoting recovery and are now commonly supplemented with "harm reduction" services intended to reduce the damage of ongoing drug use to the individual concerned as well as people around them. The concept of harm reduction is familiar to anyone who has seen an advertising campaign against drunk driving. Such public service advertisements don't tell people not to drink; rather they encourage people to change other behavior in the hopes that alcohol use will thereby become less harmful.

Many people wonder why health professionals would provide sterile injecting equipment to someone who is addicted to injectable drugs, vaccinate them against hepatitis B they could contract with continued needle sharing, or give out a medication that doesn't stop people from using heroin but could save their life if they overdose from using it. After all, isn't the goal to stop people from using the drug to which they are addicted rather than facilitating it? Clearly, the best outcome for someone who is, say, injecting heroin several times a day is never to use heroin in any form ever again. However, there are many situations where the person is unwilling to attempt to stop using heroin or keeps trying and is not able to do so. The goal thus moves to reducing the harm of their heroin use, and sterile needles and vaccinations make it less likely that they will contract or transmit infectious disease, and naloxone makes it less likely they will get brain damage from an overdose. This is an imperfect solution, but as the adage has it, half a loaf is better than none. This argument has moved diverse people in support of harm reduction interventions, from left-wing figures such as South African Archbishop Desmond Tutu to conservative policymakers like UK Prime Minister Margaret Thatcher.

Some critics of such approaches would argue that by making drug use safer, one is extending a person's drug use career by removing a motivation for stopping, or, making people who are addicted to a drug feel more comfortable transitioning to more risky forms of use (e.g., injecting). Such concerns have a rational basis—people drive faster when they wear their seat belts because they feel safer, for example—but the added health harm that is caused by some people responding to harm reduction interventions by increased risky behavior is likely less than the benefit a larger number of drug users experience by receiving the intervention. One in 10 people extending their heroin use career by a year because of needle exchange is a smaller cost than, say, 3 of those 10 people contracting or transmitting an infectious disease they otherwise would not have.

Syringe exchange. Anti-drunk-driving programs are probably the most familiar form of harm reduction. For drugs other than alcohol, the best known is probably syringe exchange for people who inject drugs. Sharing needles is a common way to contract or to transmit infectious diseases like HIV and Hepatitis B and C. Syringe exchange programs make this less likely by giving out sterile equipment and taking in used needles (this also lowers the chance of a needle stick by someone walking through the park, for example).

Syringe exchange has never been subjected to a randomized trial. That said, evidence from practice and observational studies is encouraging. Injection drug users do in fact access syringe exchange programs when they are available, are more inclined after contact to use clean equipment, and also sometimes eventually use them as a portal to further health services. Studies at the community level suggest that this translates into lower rates of HIV transmission and infection among intravenous drug users. These effects likely extend benefit beyond them as well, in that a lower rate of HIV among people who use drugs should translate into a lower rate among their sexual partners whether those individuals use drugs or not.

Naloxone distribution. Naloxone is a fast-acting "antagonist" medication that binds tightly at the same receptor in the brain as do opioids, kicking opioids out of the receptor in the process. Administering naloxone does not remove the person's addiction, but does usually reverse the ability of the opioid the person has taken to stop their breathing. Broadly distributing naloxone (e.g., making it available without a prescription, having first responders carry it) and teaching people how and when to use it is an increasingly common harm reduction strategy.

There are good signs in science and in practice that naloxone reduces fatal overdose. Many people with little or no medical training are able to learn how to safely administer the medication and also to engage in the other rescue behaviors for someone experiencing opioid overdose such as cardiopulmonary resuscitation, calling an ambulance, and putting the individual into a physical position that facilitates breathing. There are no randomized clinical trials of naloxone distribution and education, but one study found that in communities where more people participated in naloxone training the opioid overdose rate was lower than in communities where fewer people learned how to recognize and respond to an overdose.

Fentanyl test strips and drug checking services. Illicit drug producers are more likely than licit producers to mislabel their products, for example, to call a pressed fentanyl pill an Atavan, or to "cut" drugs with other materials to reduce costs. Some services have grown up to help users to more reliably know the content of drugs they plan to take. Drug checking services, for example at musical festivals, allow people to present illicitly produced drugs for chemical analysis by technicians. Fentanyl test strips allow the individual themselves to determine whether or not drugs they have purchased include this potent opioid.

The idea that drugs present risk only because people don't know what they are taking is false. Many people overdose every day from clearly labeled, uncontaminated drugs, including pharmaceutical opioids, benzodiazepines, and alcohol. Also, knowledge that a drug is adulterated will not necessarily sway the use of many addicted individuals, particularly if they are in acute withdrawal. For the subset of unusually planful, well-organized people who are addicted to drugs, there may be some benefit to drug checking interventions, though at the population level any benefit would be small.

Overall, the evidence for harm reduction interventions has always been and likely always will be weaker than that for treatments. Harm reduction interventions are challenging to study. They cannot, for example, be randomly assigned to patients in controlled settings to judge their efficacy under easily studied conditions. Harm reduction tends to happen at the community level with populations that are difficult to track and interventions that are difficult to standardize. A harm reduction worker who gives away 10,000 fentanyl test strips in a community hopes that those who take them use them to prevent overdoses, but may never know if and how often this happened.

On the other hand, some harm reduction interventions are inexpensive to deliver and easily scalable. This means they can cover a significant swathe of the addicted population in a way a more intensive clinical intervention never could. From this viewpoint, even if the impact on most people who receive interventions is nil and for the rest it is only small, there could still be a net population public health benefit. Also, pragmatically speaking, for the population who are addicted to drugs and have no interest in quitting, it's harm reduction or nothing at all, so even a small benefit can beat the alternative.

There's another point to remember if one believes the only legitimate function of services is to reduce substance use. Although harm reduction isn't in the philosophical abstract intended to reduce drug use, as a practical matter when addicted people become engaged with some service that is attempting to help them change their health behavior, they usually in fact reduce the amount of their drug use anyway. Likewise, some people who seek "abstinence focused" addiction treatment end up continuing to use drugs but nonetheless lower their risk. In other areas of health care, mixing and matching treatments focused on curing illnesses versus managing them is so routine that no one even thinks to divide them into "treatment" and "harm reduction." This should be accepted as a reality in the care of people experiencing addiction.

Peer-led supports for recovery

Addiction treatment is organized by paid and licensed physicians, psychologists, nurses, social workers, and other individuals trained in the science and practice of caring for patients. This system exists in parallel with voluntary systems of support outside the health care system which are organized and operated by individuals who have personal experience of addiction, generally from experiencing it themselves but also including individuals otherwise affected by it. Such initiatives form an important part of the de facto care system for addiction in many countries.

Mutual help groups. Despite the enormous effort that governments and individual professionals put into standing up and staffing all the treatment services just described, the most common settings in which addicted people seek help around the world are not run by professionals at all. Rather they are peer-led mutual help groups (also sometimes called "self-help groups," "mutual aid groups," or "fellowships").

Mutual help groups for addiction share some features of professional treatment in that they are devoted to helping people recover and feature some activities commonly found in treatment, for example people meeting in groups and discussing their experiences. But the similarities end there.

First, mutual help groups are not run by professionals nor licensed in any way, rather they are peer-created and -led grassroots resources. Second, the claim to expertise in mutual groups does not rest on education or other formal credentials, but on having "been there" with an addiction oneself and now being in recovery. Third, unlike treatment, mutual help groups require no paperwork, no private or public insurance payment, and charge no fees beyond small voluntary contributions. Fourth, in treatment the professional is a designated helper and the patient is a designated helpee, but in mutual help groups helping is a two-way street, that is, the same person might be in the role of helper at one moment and being helped in the next. Fifth, mutual help participation can go on indefinitely and become integrated into daily life in a fashion that treatment generally cannot. That is, mutual help is a community and way of living and being rather than a discrete professional health care service delivered for a set period in a specialized context.

The best known of mutual help organizations is Alcoholics Anonymous, which was founded by two men in the Midwest United States in the 1930s and has since become a presence in over 180 countries, with around 5 million members. AA members, who refer to themselves as "recovering alcoholics" (as opposed to "ex-alcoholics" or "recovered" alcoholics), meet in groups that they run themselves, and in which they offer each other "experience, strength, and hope" that facilitates recovery. AA groups are easy to attend (no appointments required, no fees) as well as easy to start. Any two members can found a new AA meeting because, for example, they want a non-smoking meeting, one focused on a particular population (e.g., women, people with comorbid psychiatric problems, gay/lesbian, Spanish speaking), or one that is simply more practically convenient for them (e.g., in a part of town or time of day which currently lacks a meeting). AA's comfort with letting members found groups has helped the organization spread and also to bring support to a very diverse population.

In addition to emotional support and practical strategies to achieve and maintain sobriety, AA offers "sponsorship." A sponsor is an experienced member who guides newer members through the recovery process. AA also publishes and distributes free books and pamphlets that illuminate different aspects of its program. AA's philosophy of change is known as the "12 steps," which guide members not only to stop drinking forever but also to face up to and atone for the mistakes they have made, to relate more honestly and responsibly to people in their lives, to develop an attitude of spiritual humility, and to carry the AA message to others. Members are not in any way obligated to follow the 12 steps, but most put some weight on them.

AA's approach has been copied outright or adapted by many other mutual help organizations around the world, from The Links in Sweden to Danshukai in Japan. AA's model has also been employed for countless addictions other than alcohol. The general principles of AA have also been adapted by individuals affected by addiction, including family members of addicted individuals (e.g., Al-Anon) as well as people who were raised by them (e.g., Adult Children of Alcoholics). Some ideas from AA were also incorporated into a peer-led residential living option known as Oxford House.

AA and the organizations it inspired are the most common form of addiction-related mutual help organization. But there are alternatives. Some organizations have formed as a direct response to AA's approach, specifically trying to offer individuals something different. Moderation Management, for example, attracts people with less severe drinking problems than the typical AA member, and tries to support members in returning to less harmful drinking rather than insisting on abstinence. Women for Sobriety takes a feminist approach to recovery, restricting membership to women and emphasizing the building of self-esteem rather than the instillation of humility that is valued in AA. LifeRing Secular Recovery eschews the spiritual elements found in AA. Perhaps the most intriguing thing about all these alternatives to AA is that many and perhaps most people who attend them also attend AA, indicating that people mix and match groups that are ostensibly in philosophical conflict.

Other mutual help organizations have no connection to AA either as inspiration or as counter-inspiration. France, for example, has Vie Libre, an alcohol mutual help organization that grew out of workers' union movements, and many Indigenous communities in the US have recovery supporting organizations they have created on their own. These and many other examples of mutual help organizations around the world suggest that there is something in the experience of addiction that leads many people to conclude that a community of fellow sufferers can help them find recovery.

Policymakers, clinicians, and individuals seeking recovery are naturally interested in whether mutual help groups are effective. Evaluating mutual help groups in randomized clinical trials is challenging because they are not controlled by professionals. For example, although a new medication can be withheld from the control group in a treatment study, there is no way to stop the "controls" from going to mutual help groups on their own in a study of AA or Women for Sobriety or any other mutual help group. That mutual help organizations generally value anonymity and do not track members over time creates further challenges.

However, multiple rigorous studies have been conducted which support the effectiveness of Alcoholics Anonymous and some other mutual help models as well (e.g., Oxford Houses). The most rigorous integration of the best AA research was a Cochrane Collaboration review that showed AA and 12-step facilitation counseling were more effective than high-quality professionally provided treatments for achieving abstinence and just as effective for achieving other outcomes (e.g., reduced drinking-related consequences and drinks per drinking day). The same review also showed that AA, which is free to attend, reduces members' use of health care services, thereby saving society substantial money.

Mutual help groups are tailor made for enhancing one type of outcome, namely rebuilding a healthy social network. When they enter addiction treatment, many patients are in the habit of spending much of their time with other individuals who heavily use substances, which makes it harder to sustain recovery. Mutual help groups provide an unusually easy way to "swap out" substance-using friends with non-using friends, and the evidence indicates that many members find this important in early recovery. They also provide a chance to build a social network from scratch for patients whose friends and family have disowned them.

Other recovery supportive resources. People in recovery from addiction have become more organized and more vocal in recent decades, which has helped to lower cultural stigma toward addiction, advance the rights of individuals who experience it, and create new forms of recovery support. One example is recovery schools, which support the education of teenagers and young adults in recovery. This is particularly important because both that time of life as well as those settings (particularly universities) are characterized by prevalent heavy substance use, which poses a risk of relapse.

Recovering community centers are non-profit organizations operating a physical club-like setting that serves as the hub for many activities, be it mutual help group meetings, friend making, advocacy training, and linkage to employment and social service resources. Recovery music and art festivals enrich the life of the recovery community in selected cities around the world. Recovery marches, which are organized in an increasing number of cities and countries, have a more activist bent, typically making demands on politicians (e.g., for better funded, more accessible treatment) while also serving to make recovery easier by reducing cultural stigma.

Faith communities are the other arena of recovery support outside of the treatment system that bears mention. A subset of mutual help organizations explicitly tie their approach to a religious framework, with Alcoholics for Christ, Calix Society, Celebrate Recovery, Millati Islami, and Jewish Alcoholics, Chemically Dependent Persons and Significant Others being examples. These organizations often meet in houses of worship and bring in more specific theology than would be the case in "spiritual" mutual help organizations that leave such matters to a wide range of individual interpretation. Expression of religious faith in such organizations is welcome more than in secular groups or those that see spiritual matters as subjectively defined. A few faith communities around the world have been composed entirely of individuals with addiction experience, though it is more common that a church, mosque, synagogue, or temple will support a subset of such individuals, for example individuals seeking recovery after leaving prison. Finally, it should be noted that clergy across many faiths provide substantial counseling to many people, including at times on the subject of addiction.

Chapter 5
Cultural and public policy approaches to addiction

Societies vary dramatically in their prevalence of addiction and in how addiction is experienced by individuals and those around them. Some of this variation is explained by the different approaches societies take to drugs and to addiction. Countries typically have formal laws, regulations, and programs focused on drugs and designed to reduce addiction, which are referred to as public policy. All societies also have something less tangible but still important, namely the widespread practices and beliefs around drugs and addiction in the population, which will be discussed here as cultural approaches.

There are cultures and subcultures that are abstemious, those that celebrate intoxication, and all manner in between. Because a person cannot become addicted without using drugs, cultures and subcultural norms regarding drug use and intoxication influence the incidence of addiction. In most Islamic countries, for example, alcohol use is subject to significant social disapproval. Such societies have very low alcohol consumption rates, and hence low rates of alcohol addiction. In contrast, British culture embraces more positive attitudes about alcohol use, and unsurprisingly has higher rates of alcohol consumption and addiction.

Cultures also vary in how much they stigmatize addiction, which is a distinct question from whether they approve of drug use;

Why are drug problems so different in Lisbon and San Francisco?

Cultural attitudes about drug use and intoxication influence the outcomes of different drug policies. Lisbon is in a country which applies no criminal penalties for drug use or possession and provides generous health and social care services to people facing addiction. In recent years, San Francisco attempted to copy Lisbon's approach but, unlike that Portuguese city, it has high rates of drug use, open air drug markets, significant drug-related disorder, and high rates of overdose, including one or more people dying on the street most days of the year.

The difference is probably cultural: San Francisco celebrates intoxication, being for decades a hub of the cannabis and psychedelic drug subcultures, and being one of the heaviest drinking cities in the US for more than a century. The "City by the Bay" also has a highly mobile population, with many people disconnected from family obligations and other social network constraints. San Francisco has a culture that is individualistic and focused on personal fulfillment as a right and even an obligation. Lisbon, in contrast, has a more communitarian culture in which obligations to others are valued more than celebration of self. Excessive drug use is disapproved of socially, even though legally it is largely tolerated. Pressuring people with addictions into treatment is seen as highly desirable. In addition to being in a more socially conservative society, Lisbon also has more long-term residents in stable social networks of connection and responsibility, including many people whose parents and grandparents also live in Lisbon.

When the curbs on drug use provided by law enforcement were relaxed in Lisbon, their robust cultural norms against it remained in place. But in San Francisco, the law was the main source of

(*continued*)

anti-intoxication norms, and when those were removed all that was left was a culture with no such restraints. Thus a public policy that looked similar on paper generated wildly different outcomes in two places with divergent cultures.

some societies valorize drug use but shun those for whom it becomes a problem. In most societies, addiction is a deeply stigmatized condition, sometimes viewed as a sign of moral failure, bad character, sinful pleasure seeking, inherent criminality, genetic inferiority, or disapproval by a deity. Through history, terms like "junkie," "meth freak," "dope fiend," and "pot head" have reflected cultural contempt of addicted people. Such stigma comes about in part because the condition is poorly understood and in part because many people have been harmed by addicted individuals and feel punitive towards them in response.

The effects of the stigma are profound, including a preference in many societies for punishment over therapeutic responses. These punishments range from the painful (public flogging, imprisonment) to the fatal. Even in societies where addiction treatment is available, it is often poorly resourced, reflecting a widely shared if unspoken belief that quality treatment is not fundamentally deserved. Stigma may help some people avoid drug use entirely, but for those who are already addicted, being seen as a parasite or freak greatly complicates the process of acknowledging the problem and asking for help. Indeed, while addicted people are often said to be "in denial" about their problems, in many cases their unwillingness to be candid is driven as much by rational fears of negative reactions as by their own psychological blind spots. Finally, cultural attitudes towards different racial, ethnic, and income groups influence their response to addiction. Addiction that evokes sympathy when experienced by a dominant racial or ethnic group may be seen as a sign of moral inferiority in an oppressed group within the same society. In the United States for example, Black Americans experiencing opioid addiction during the heroin crisis of the 1960s and 1970s were viewed less sympathetically than were the many white Americans who became addicted to pharmaceutical opioids and heroin in the 1990s and 2000s. Dominant groups may even see fostering addiction in an oppressed population as a legitimate way to pursue profit. This was the motivation behind the opium wars, which Britain fought to force China to accept opium over its objections, at great cost to the health of that country.

Public policies toward addiction

The laws and regulations that governments create affect how much addiction they experience and the consequences of those addictions to society. Sometimes these policies explicitly address addiction and at other times they don't appear to but affect the addiction situation nonetheless. Examples of the former include when a government decides that its national health service will expand coverage for alcohol addiction or when a city mayor announces a crackdown on cocaine trafficking. Examples of the latter include broad trade policies that result (intentionally or not) in expansion or restriction of the supply of addictive products (e.g., cigarettes) in a country or Internet regulations that make it easier or harder to operate on-line gambling websites.

Public policies reflect not only evidence about which drugs are more addictive or harmful than others but also cultural norms, history, and, in democracies at least, the views of voters. Although some argue that public policy should be determined entirely technocratically, as the phrase "evidence-based policy" implies is possible, in reality this is impossible because all human beings, including scientists, have subjective values and preferences that will be reflected in how society operates.

Why is the government involved in drug policy at all? A libertarian could note accurately that many products people consume do not attract the policy attention devoted to drugs. Broccoli, for example, is sold with minimal government oversight or taxation in grocery stores, farmer's markets, and booths by the side of country roads in agricultural regions. Consumers are generally trusted to buy whatever amount and type of broccoli they need. What then is the rationale for not taking the same approach to methamphetamine or fentanyl? Why interfere in any way with the right of free people to produce, sell, purchase, and consume addictive drugs as they do broccoli?

One reason this libertarian perspective has never commanded a wide following among the public is that drug use and addiction have, as described in detail earlier in this book, large negative externalities. Unfettered use of drugs leads many people to engage in behavior that impinges on the rights of others, such as verbal and physical aggression, impaired driving, and theft. Some restrictions on the rights of people to use drugs thus have democratic support because doing so protects the rights of people who may be harmed by others' drug use.

Second, the underlying logic of free markets is that individuals can judge best for themselves what is valuable. But this assumption doesn't hold for addiction, during which impaired judgment is a central problem. Because in addiction people will sacrifice their health, family, community, values—and not incidentally their freedom—in order to keep using drugs, standing back and saying "Well, they must know best" is at best naive and at worst cruel.

Third, eliminating government action regarding drugs would not create a libertarian state-of-nature culture with no one trying to influence individuals' drug use. Because consumption of addictive substances is steeply skewed, drug producers have potent economic incentives to addict as many individuals as possible. Strategies industries pursue to accomplish this include making products stronger, more available, and more widely advertised. Individual choices under such conditions are not made free of external influence. When government intervenes with drug policy, it can make individuals more free by countering powerful commercial forces trying to shape the populations' decisions about drugs for their own purposes.

Prohibitions. A prohibition is, simply put, a law saying that some or all of the population is not allowed to do one or more activities related to drugs. These prohibitions can usefully be divided into those focused on the production and sale of drugs and those focused on the possession and use of drugs. Governments sometimes have only one of these two types of prohibitions, at other times both, and very commonly governments vary this policy mix across different drugs.

Prohibitions against the production and sale of particular drugs are common worldwide, and indeed almost all nations are signatories to United Nations treaties committing them to make production of multiple drugs (e.g., methamphetamine, cocaine, heroin) for non-medical reasons illegal. These prohibitions have a large effect because without legal corporate power behind them, drugs have a hard time gaining a foothold—alcohol and cigarettes are by far more widely used and cause more death than all illegal drugs put together because deep-pocketed legal corporations can produce, advertise, and distribute them. Likewise, the North American opioid epidemic started by legal pharmaceutical companies spread addiction far more efficiently throughout the population than any illegal opioid cartel could ever accomplish.

Prohibitions on production and sale allow interdiction of drugs by law enforcement. Sometimes, arrests and seizures produce only transitory reductions in drug use and death. But there are exceptions. For example, major law enforcement operations in Australia appeared to produce an extended "heroin drought" in the country in the 2000s. This produced a remarkable 60 percent decline in overdose deaths that lasted for many years.

Prohibitions on production and sale don't just affect drugs and drug use. Preventing the development of corporations has economic effects that some view as objectionable, that is, the government is stopping people from acquiring wealth by producing and selling a lucrative product. Some of the most vocal critics of prohibitions are extremely rich people who have made a fortune in other industries and do not see why similar fortunes shouldn't be made in the drug trade. Some people of more modest means do not have such avaricious aspirations, but would note correctly that illegal industries do not pay taxes nor create legal employment opportunities. If expanding corporate profit were humanity's only goal, legalizing all drug production and sale as well as use by any person of any age would be the most sensible policy. But because most people believe that unlimited accrual of money is not as important as preserving human life, health, and well-being, such a policy is unlikely to ever be adopted.

Many legal prohibitions around drugs are intended to reduce population exposure only to some extent. In the US, producing and selling recreational cannabis is legal in a number of states, but only if the customers are over the age of 21. Likewise, most countries with legal alcohol have a drinking age under which alcohol purchase and consumption are not permitted. The focus of many prohibitions on youth use follows from cultural beliefs about vulnerability as well as evolved habits of parents wanting to protect their offspring. These beliefs and impulses have a rational root. Neuroscientific research shows that young brains are far more "plastic" (i.e., changeable, adaptable) than older brains. Acquiring an addiction is easier for the young than old, much as is acquiring fluency in a foreign language. This helps explain why almost all addictions begin when individuals are young (i.e., under the age of 25) and why societies try to prohibit use of and marketing of drugs to youth.

Another form of partial prohibition centers on medical versus non-medical uses of drugs. Many drugs that can be harmful, such as cocaine and hydrocodone, also can be helpful to patients receiving health care. Most societies grapple with this duality by applying a partial prohibition to such drugs: producing them for recreational use is illegal, but producing them for health care systems that will prescribe them in medical practice is legal. Advocates for reduced prohibitions often argue their case by claiming that certain drugs (e.g., cannabis, psychedelic mushrooms) have miraculous medical benefits even when the evidence for such claims is scanty.

Another type of legal prohibition targets not drug use per se but its harm. Anti-impaired driving laws forbid drug use (e.g., consuming alcohol and cannabis) only while driving. Other such laws include making it illegal to operate heavy equipment at a worksite, use firearms in the military or the police, fly a commercial airplane, drive a school bus, or perform surgery under the influence of drugs. Such prohibitions, typically backed up by biological tests, have substantial evidence of reducing harm from substance use. Although not their primary purpose, they may also result in some people using drugs less, for example the person who offers to become the designated driver for guests at a boozy party.

Other prohibitions are location based. In order to protect employees, many countries and cities ban smoking of tobacco and cannabis in the workplace including restaurants and bars. "Open container" laws preventing drinking in public areas are another example.

Prohibitions also can apply to the person who uses a drug. In some countries, drug use per se is prohibited, whereas in others the possession of drugs with presumed intent to use is the focus of prohibition. Many but certainly not all countries apply less severe prohibitions to users of drugs than they do to those who produce and sell them. The sentencing guidelines applied under the UK Misuse of Drugs Act, for example, recommend more severe punishments (e.g., imprisonment) for those who manufacture drugs than those who use them.

To have a prohibition means to enforce a prohibition. The types of penalties applied may be criminal (e.g., arrest and/or incarceration) or civil (e.g., cautions and fines). Penalties can help deter some individuals from breaking the prohibition. They also—except in the case of fines that are generally paid—cost money to enforce. Further, the harms done by punishments can exceed those done by the drugs themselves, particularly for already oppressed groups in a society.

Finally, by definition, prohibiting something increases crime, because once a law is created in any domain, at least some people will break it. It may seem to follow from this observation that prohibition is the cause of the association of drugs with crime. Yet, as mentioned earlier, alcohol, which is legal for adults to consume in most societies, is a far bigger contributor to crime, arrests, and incarceration than all prohibited drugs put together. Although prohibition creates criminals, it also reduces drug use dramatically, which reduces intoxication-fueled crime. So if cocaine were legalized like alcohol, no one who used or sold cocaine per se would be defined as a criminal. But with legal companies able to produce and market it, cocaine consumption would increase, which would increase crime because some cocaine users would engage in behavior (especially aggression and extreme risk-taking) they otherwise would not do.

Regulation of addiction producing industries. As mentioned, addiction producing industries almost always are shaped by a partial prohibition against selling the product to youth. Beyond that, most countries subject these industries to forms of regulation that can change the prevalence of addiction as well as have other effects, including raising revenue for the government.

The most prevalent example is taxes, which raise the price of the addictive product beyond what it would be in a free market, sometimes considerably so. Taxes never raise the price of a drug as much as does forbidding its production and sale, but can certainly raise it sufficiently to lessen use. This is particularly true in "price-sensitive" populations, for example adolescents who don't have much pocket money.

Critics of increased taxes on drugs sometimes argue that "Addicted people will do anything to get their drug." This is wrong-headed in two ways. First, policies such as raising taxes on cigarettes have their primary benefit in discouraging non-addicted people from taking up the habit in the first place. Second, abundant research shows that addicted people are sensitive to cost. When prices rise, even addicted individuals consume less of a drug. This principle applies to financial cost as well as to search time, risk of punishment, and social disapproval. As an example of the latter, addicted smokers do not light up during religious services even where such behavior is legal, and smoking on commercial airplane flights is equally rare even though hundreds of millions of tobacco-addicted individuals fly each year.

Another class of regulation focuses on marketing of drugs, for example making it illegal to advertise cigarettes or alcohol on children's television programs. Reducing such cues not only may reduce the likelihood of people initiating use but also could help those with existing addictions to not use as much or to sustain a recovery attempt.

Regulations can also limit the availability of drugs in many other ways. Requiring a license for sale lowers the number of retail outlets, as can zoning laws preventing businesses from operating in residential areas or near schools. For some drugs, including liquor in Sweden and cannabis in the Canadian province of Quebec, another way to limit availability is to have the government itself operate retail outlets. Research in many nations has shown that reducing availability of sales outlets lowers drug use and related problems.

Providing services to people facing addiction. The previous chapter described a range of health and social care services that help people experiencing addiction or on the path to doing so. The availability and type of these services do not arise at random, but are a function of the public policy environment.

In some countries, addiction treatment is not considered part of health care policy. This generally results in support for people seeking recovery coming entirely from the voluntary sector, for example charities, religious organizations, and peer-led resources. Some of these organizations offer high quality assistance, and their informal nature may make them more comfortable to access than, say, hospitals. But the voluntary sector often lacks the capacity of health care systems, particularly in terms of offering treatment for co-occurring problems like infectious disease and psychotic disorders.

Other countries frame addiction treatment as a part of criminal justice policy. This was initially the case in the post-war US, when the federal government built "narcotics farms" in Fort Worth, Texas and Lexington, Kentucky. These facilities were intended to treat addiction, but were operated by the Federal Bureau of Prisons and "patients" were sentenced to them rather than being able to come and go if they wished. Other countries have similar arrangements today. For example in China and Vietnam addicted individuals are sent off for years to what are called "camps" but are for all practical purposes correctional facilities with few therapeutic services. Crudely put, the logic of such approaches is to send the person far away and "knock some sense into them." In addition to potentially imperiling the human rights of addicted people, there is no evidence of such approaches helping people enter recovery. Afterwards people return to their communities, facing the same problems that were there before and with no ongoing support, and, potentially traumatized by their "treatment." This is not a good basis for recovery from addiction.

In wealthier countries, addiction treatment is usually considered within health care policy. This can bring significant budgetary resources to the enterprise as well as reach into different populations and geographic areas. It can also reduce the stigma of services by nesting them in a system with significant social trust in which patients feel comfortable, that is, asking one's trusted doctor for advice about drug use is easier than walking straight into an "addiction treatment agency" across town.

That said, countries (and regions within countries) vary enormously in how much they resource addiction care within health. In many countries, addiction treatment commands a smaller share of health care budgets than would seem justified by the toll addiction takes on population health. In the US, for example, for many years it was legal for private health insurance plans to set benefits for addiction care lower than care for any other condition. This was also true in government insurance programs: When Medicare was created in the US, it covered 80 percent of outpatient health care bills, except for addiction and mental health care, for which it only covered 50 percent. It took substantial advocacy to change these policies. Countries sometimes lurch between neglecting and investing in addiction treatment based on whether the problem is at a crisis stage or not. The United Kingdom spent a decade steadily cutting funding for drug addiction treatment until a greatly deteriorating situation led government to massively reinvest in it beginning in 2021.

Preventing addiction

As this book has made clear, addiction does great harm to those who experience it, their families, and society as a whole. Treating addiction is therefore a noble goal, but it would obviously be even better to prevent people from becoming addicted in the first place. Public policies can have a significant impact in this area.

When we ask what can be done to prevent a problem like addiction, we sometimes mix the question of what can be done in general for the population and what can be done for any one person. For instance, untreated mental illness might explain why a particular person in a city is homeless (therefore providing more treatment for mental illness would seem to prevent homelessness), but the reason why anyone at all is homeless in the city could be that rents have risen much faster than wages. Untreated mental illness only determines who doesn't have a chair when the music stops playing, not the shortage of chairs per se.

With addiction we therefore must distinguish what can be done to prevent any one person from becoming addicted (including you or a loved one if that is why you are reading this book) and what can be done for addiction in the population as a whole. Science teaches much more about the latter question than the former.

Preventing addiction in individuals. Beyond the obvious advice to individuals that if you don't use a drug in the first place, you can't become addicted to it, there are no guarantees for individuals who hope to avoid addiction. That is, for example, you can be born with genes that make the average person's risk of addiction lower, participate in prevention programs that benefit the average person, live in a society with supply control policies that reduce the overall population rate of drug use, yet still end up being addicted to a drug. Individual lives are simply hard to predict. This is particularly important to remember if you are the parent of a child who develops a drug addiction. Many parents assume they somehow caused their child's addiction, and that if they had just parented differently it would not have happened. Parenting of course does influence children, yet probably every clinician in the addiction field has encountered young people who grew up with devoted, competent, non-addicted parents yet developed an addiction anyway.

It is a bit anxiety producing to realize that beyond the principle that you can't get addicted to a drug you never use, science can't predict very accurately who will become addicted. This reality should also generate compassion. Most people will use drugs at some point in their lives, whether recreationally, medically, or both. If scientists can't guess after decades of research which of those individuals will become addicted and which will not, it's safe to assume that those individuals can't do so either. When you meet an addicted person, remember that there are other people who used precisely the same drugs as they did yet did not become addicted, and this difference is heavily influenced by factors we don't yet understand. People who progress to addiction are not inherently morally worse than people who use drugs without becoming addicted; they could just be less lucky due to genes, environments, life experiences, and other factors no one can fully control.

Reducing the incidence of addiction in the population. In contrast to preventing addiction in any given individual, science does know a significant amount about how to reduce the overall incidence of addiction in the population. Turning scientific knowledge into effective prevention policies requires focusing on the subset of predictive factors that are changeable.

For example, as has been discussed, particular genes can increase risk for addiction, and the working of the human brain can be altered by repeated drug consumption to cause addiction. But at a population level, neither of these facts is very useful for prevention policy. Short of a eugenics program that would be morally objectionable to almost anyone, the genes of the population are what they are. Likewise, the human brain has evolved over tens of thousands of years. It took a long time to become what it is and it's not getting better anytime soon.

Thus, paradoxically, understanding genetics and neuroscience should lead us to think about what has changed much more in recent decades and what we have much more power to change again: the environment. No one can get addicted without using drugs, so it follows that limiting exposure to drugs in the environment is a potent way to reduce the prevalence of addiction in the population.

Previous chapters discussed many ways to accomplish this, including prohibiting production and sale of drugs, partially prohibiting drugs (e.g., for children and adolescents), and tightly regulating the tobacco, cannabis, alcohol, and gambling industries to make their products harder to access. Because enforcing laws and regulations is typically done by the criminal justice system, many people overlook that all of these approaches are fundamentally public health strategies, just as much as reducing bacteria in the water supply is part of the public health approach for reducing population disease.

Drug supply control and corporate regulation covers whole regions and populations. Other prevention efforts cover subsets of the population. One of them is testing people for substance use at their worksite, with some consequence for a positive test. When the US military instituted drug testing with penalties up to and including expulsion, drug use promptly dropped by 80 percent. Likewise, professions with regular testing, such as airplane pilots, have lower rates of substance use disorders. That said, drug testing in schools has not generated comparable results, perhaps because it is harder to implement at scale in an effective and fair fashion.

Other prevention programs rely on persuasion, education, and skill building to attempt to reduce the incidence of addiction. These programs are usually targeted at young people and are delivered in educational settings. The best known of these programs is, perhaps unfortunately, Drug Abuse Resistance

Education (DARE) which sent police officers into schools to provide information about drugs and discourage children from using them. DARE has repeatedly been shown to have poor evidence of effectiveness (though after multiple stem-to-stern revisions, its latest incarnation seems to have some modest benefit).

More effective programs focus, perhaps surprisingly, less on specific beliefs and intentions about drugs and more on children's environment, and generic skills and capacities that young people need to thrive across many domains. Environmentally focused programs include those that restructure classrooms to reward positive behavior and group cooperation, as well as those that strengthen the connection of children with families and civic and cultural groups.

Generic skill programs instill capacities such as recognizing and managing emotions, gaining self-control, and relating positively to other people. Generic skill and capacity building programs recognize that the risk factors for young people becoming addicted overlap with virtually every other problem for which youth are at risk, such as depression, self-harm, school dropout, bullying, and social isolation. A successful program that embraces this strategy, Communities that Care, showed evidence of reducing young people's use of tobacco, alcohol, and other drugs, and also had radiating benefits in terms of reducing delinquent behavior and violence and increasing prosocial ties.

Chapter 6
The future of addiction

The landscape of addiction in humans has changed more in the past two centuries than in the tens of thousands of years before that. It would be foolish therefore to expect that this rapid rate of change will cease. A number of important trends are already evident.

The rise of synthetic drugs

For most of human history, humanity's use of drugs was restricted to naturally occurring or lightly processed molecules found in nature. Startling advances in technology and chemistry changed this situation dramatically beginning in the 19th century, and this continues today, not just in high-end laboratories but also in many a kitchen sink. Synthetic addictive drugs are becoming more prevalent due to the decreasing costs of the required equipment and chemicals, more widespread education (e.g., in chemistry), and the ease of sharing drug production strategies over the Internet.

From the point of view of illicit drug traffickers, the attractions of synthetic drugs are many. Not needing plants to make drugs means not needing to find arable land and people to farm it in politically volatile areas. Traffickers are also freed of concerns about drought and crop blight, and about interdiction of multi-ton shipments of drugs somewhere in globe spanning supply chains.

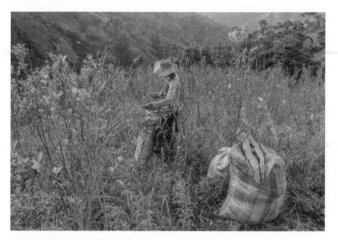

5. Farming coca to make cocaine could become a thing of the past if synthetic drugs proliferate.

Instead drugs can be made indoors by small teams, come rain or shine. And production can be based close to retail markets, reducing the risk of an interdiction at sea or at a border inspection.

The rise of synthetic drugs poses great challenges to traditional approaches to drug control that focus on drug crops in faraway lands (Figure 5). If this makes supply control policies less effective, it would increase availability of drugs and therefore, as we have discussed, the rate of addiction.

The unknown factor when it comes to synthetic drugs is whether, as chemistry techniques and knowledge of neuroscience advance, drugs can be designed to be even more addictive. This could be done by increasing their positive reinforcement value or by eliminating their negative effects (e.g., by designing an ethanol molecule that didn't produce a hangover). The economic incentives to do this are large, so chemists will definitely try their hand at producing such drugs.

On the other hand, increased ability to manipulate the molecular structure of drugs could make iatrogenic addiction less common. Opioids, for example, simultaneously activate brain pathways that reduce pain, cause euphoria, and slow breathing. Animal research suggests the action of these pathways can be separated. For example, if science developed an opioid painkiller that provided analgesia but not euphoria, it would be less addicting. Or if it developed an opioid that did not reduce rate of breathing, it would mean doctors could treat pain patients with less risk of overdose, and that addicted individuals could be more protected from overdose as well (e.g., in methadone maintenance treatment).

Increased tailoring of addictive products

The ability of purveyors of addiction to become more effective in the future by tailoring their wares is not limited to biochemistry. Computers and artificial intelligence are already allowing an expansion of addiction to gambling. Electronic slot machines eclipse their mechanical forebears ("one-armed bandits") in their unrivalled ability to provide reinforcement at just the right rates and speed to instill addiction. In some communities, this has already produced near epidemic levels of financial ruin from these machines.

Every company that develops a video game, app, social media site, or the like wants it to be "addictive" and the ability to achieve this will increase over time. Because at least some people are willing even to have implants or wires attached during their virtual experiences, one could even imagine a perfectly designed system that is more satisfying to some people than daily life ever could be.

New addiction treatments

Because addiction is a complex, chronic, behaviorally embedded disorder, it may prove no easier to treat in the future than it is today. But at least some breakthroughs are possible. Some studies have shown that providing direct stimulation to particular regions in the brain helps addicted people recover. Most commonly, these interventions target the dorsolateral prefrontal cortex, a region of the forebrain which is associated with executive control (e.g., working memory, attention allocation, forethought, and impulse control). The findings are inconsistent, in part because studies examine different addictions and use different methods of providing neurostimulation (e.g., ultrasound, transcranial magnetic stimulation), but like many medical technologies this one could advance over time.

A much more invasive approach would be putting stimulation devices directly into brains. Only one person has successfully undergone this procedure thus far, but it could become more common. It will likely be limited only to severe cases of addiction which have not responded to other treatments, given both the costs and risks of the procedure.

As was the case in the late 1960s, some people are enthusiastic about the possibility that psychedelic drugs can cure addiction. In the initial wave of such work, the hype was crushed by the data, but better formulation methods and stronger evaluation designs could reveal new therapies of this form.

Corporate control and regulation

Perhaps nothing will shape the future of addiction more than the extent to which producing and supplying addictive drugs is allowed to flourish as an economic activity. The deadliest future would see the wealthiest 1 percent of the population manage to convince voters and policymakers to let multinational corporations sell all addictive drugs—methamphetamine, heroin, cocaine—as they now sell alcohol and tobacco. Given the health and safety harms caused by just those two currently legal drugs, it is hard to calculate how many more deaths would result from legalization of corporate production of all drugs, but perhaps drugs would collectively become the dominant contributors to death in our species.

Such a system would also accelerate inequality to levels beyond any that modern societies have seen. Broadly speaking, the profits of legal drug sales flow to the wealthy from the poor, but their ability to accentuate inequality goes beyond that purely economic reality. A complete corporate takeover of drug production could coexist with a political system in which the masses toiled on behalf of the rich, much like the cannibalistic Morlocks did for the Eloi in H. G. Wells's *The Time Machine*. But while the Eloi had to fear the Morlocks' appetites, in the darkest possible future those at the bottom of society would be pacified and kept subservient via a steady diet of transitory reinforcement from cannabis, alcohol, and other drugs, perhaps as well as on-line games and pornography.

A more positive future would be for the public to demand and politicians to comply with tighter regulations of addictive products and the corporations that supply them, on the grounds that the wealth they generate for a small number of people is not worth the damage they inflict on tens of millions of others. Combined with an expansion of effective health and social services for people experiencing addiction, this could create a future in which the toll of addiction was lessened. Whether societies get to this brighter future is a question of political will, but an understanding of the nature of addiction is also essential. I hope this book has equipped readers with such understanding, so that they can make intelligent and compassionate choices for themselves, their families, and the societies in which they live.

References

Chapter 1: Understanding the terrain

Poe's description of why he used drugs is in a letter he wrote to Sarah Whitman, which she quotes in her book *Edgar Poe and His Critics* (New York: Rudd & Carleton, 1860).

Cherie Currie's description of her drug addiction appears in her autobiography, co-authored with Tony O'Neill, *Neon Angel: A Memoir of a Runaway* (New York: It Books, 2011).

The work of James Olds and Peter Milner is described in their paper "Positive reinforcement produced by electrical stimulation of the septal area and other regions of rat brain," *Journal of Comparative and Physiological Psychology*, 47, pp. 19–27 (1954).

Chapter 2: The nature of addiction

The quote by Thomas Trotter can be found in *An Essay, Medical Philosophical, and Chemical, on Drunkenness and Its Effects on the Human Body* (London: Longman, Hurst, Rees & Orme, 1804). Further details on his life and thinking are in B. Vale and G. Edwards, *Physician to the Fleet: The Life and Times of Thomas Trotter, 1760–1832* (London: Boydell & Brewer, 2011).

L. Davies, *Candy: A Novel of Love and Addiction* (New York: Ballantine Books, 1998).

P. D. Schüll, *Addiction by Design: Machine Gambling in Las Vegas* (Princeton: Princeton University Press, 2012).

Epidemiological data on national substance use is available on-line from many sources, including the UK Office of National Statistics, the US National Survey on Drug Use and Health, and the

European Monitoring Center for Drugs and Drug Addiction. Another useful source is H. Ritchie and M. Roser, *Our World in Data: Drug Use, 2019*. Available on-line at <https://ourworldindata.org/drug-use>.

The importance of not scolding people for being resistant to the idea that addiction is a disease is elaborated in K. Humphreys, "How to deliver a more persuasive message regarding addiction as a medical disorder," *Journal of Addiction Medicine*, pp. 174–5 (2017).

M. Lowry, *Under the Volcano* (New York: Harper, 1947).

The argument that addiction is a chronic illness akin to diabetes, asthma, and hypertension was made in A. T. McLellan, D. C. Lewis, C. P. O'Brien, and H. D. Kleber, "Drug dependence, a chronic medical illness: Implications for treatment, insurance, and outcomes evaluation," *JAMA*, 284, pp. 1689–95 (2000).

A. Hasan, R. von Keller, C. M. Friemel, W. Hall, M. Schneider, D. Koethe, F. M. Leweke, W. Strube, and E. Hoch, "Cannabis use and psychosis: a review of reviews," *European Archives of Psychiatry and Clinical Neuroscience*, pp. 403–12 (2020).

Chapter 3: Causes of addiction

Data on the rise and role of the tobacco industry comes from R. Proctor, *Golden Holocaust: Origins of the Cigarette Catastrophe and the Case for Abolition* (Berkeley: University of California Press, 2012).

An analysis of the rise of the North American opioid crisis and corporations' role in fomenting it is available in K. Humphreys, C. L. Shover, C. M. Andrews, A. S. B. Bohnert, M. L. Brandeau, J. P. Caulkins, J. H. Chen, M.-F. Cuéllar, Y. L. Hurd, D. N. Juurlink, H. K. Koh, E. E. Krebs, A. Lembke, S. C. Mackey, L. L. Ouellette, B. Suffoletto, and C. Timko, "Responding to the opioid crisis in North America and beyond: Recommendations of the Stanford-Lancet Commission," *Lancet*, 399, pp. 555–604 (2022).

Data on religious influences on substance use can be found in K. Humphreys and E. Gifford, "Religion, spirituality and the troublesome use of substances". In W. R. Miller and K. Carroll (eds), *Rethinking Substance Abuse: What the Science Shows and What we should Do about it* (pp. 257–74) (New York: Guilford, 2006).

B. K. Alexander, R. B. Coambs, and P. F. Hadaway, "The effect of housing and gender on morphine self-administration in rats," *Psychopharmacology*, 58, pp. 175–9 (1978).

A. Lembke, "Time to abandon the self-medication hypothesis in patients with psychiatric disorders," *The American Journal of Drug and Alcohol Abuse*, 38/6, pp. 524–9 (2012).

The quote by William S. Burroughs is in his book, *Junkie: Confessions of an Unredeemed Drug Addict* (New York: Ace Books, 1953).

Data on young drinking problems and societal inequality can be found in D. Cameron and R. McKechnie, "Thoughts and some data on The Spirit Level", *New Directions in the Study of Alcohol*, 35, pp. 21–4 (2013). See also R. Bentley et al., "Alcohol and tobacco consumption: What is the role of economic security," *Addiction*, 116, pp. 1882–91 (2021).

Data on genetic risk for addiction and on how family history influences the subjective effects of drugs can be found in M. A. Schuckit, "A brief history of research on the genetics of alcohol and other drug use disorders," *Journal of Studies on Alcohol and Drugs*, 75/ (Suppl 17), pp. 59–67 (2014).

Chapter 4: Recovery and treatment

Hannah's story of recovery is in the public domain and can be accessed at <https://ryanhampton.org/im-willing-to-do-anything-to-stay-on-my-sober-journey/>. The website also includes many other personal stories of addiction and recovery.

G. E. Vaillant, *The Natural History of Alcoholism Revisited* (2nd edition) (Cambridge, MA: Harvard University Press, 1985).

Data on national recovery rates can be found in J. W. Kelly, B. G. Bergman, B. Hoeppner, C. Vilsaint, and W. L. White, "Prevalence and pathways of recovery from drug and alcohol problems in the United States population: Implications for practice, research, and policy," *Drug and Alcohol Dependence*, 181, pp. 162–9 (2017).

K. Humphreys, *Circles of Recovery: Self-Help Organisations for Addictions* (Cambridge: Cambridge University Press, 2004).

An accessible introduction to contingency management in addiction treatment is provided in S. T. Higgins and N. M. Petry, "Contingency management: Incentives for sobriety," *Alcohol Research and Health*, 23, pp. 122–7 (1999).

Extensive findings on the 24/7 Sobriety program are available at <https://www.rand.org/health-care/projects/24–7.html>.

J. F. Kelly, K. Humphreys, and M. Ferri, "Alcoholics Anonymous and other 12-step programs for alcohol use disorder," *Cochrane*

Database of Systematic Reviews, Issue 3. Art. No.: CD012880.
DOI: 10.1002/14651858.CD012880.pub2. (2020).

A. Y. Walley, Z. Xuan, H. H. Hackman, E. Quinn, M. Doe-Simkins,
A. Sorensen-Alawad, S. Ruiz, and A. Ozonoff, "Opioid overdose
rates and implementation of overdose education and nasal
naloxone distribution in Massachusetts: interrupted time series
analysis," *British Medical Journal*, 346:f174. doi: 10.1136/bmj.f174
(Jan. 30 2013).

Chapter 5: Cultural and public policy approaches to addiction

For a discussion of what science can and cannot provide to the
formation of public policy, see K. Humphreys and P. Piot,
"Scientific evidence alone is not sufficient basis for health policy,"
British Medical Journal, 344, e1316 (2012).

Extensive description of evidence-based prevention programs can be
found in chapter 5 of the *U.S. Surgeon General's Report on Alcohol,
Drugs, and Health*. Available on-line at <https://addiction.
surgeongeneral.gov/>.

T. Babor et al., *Drug Policy and the Public Good* (Oxford: Oxford
University Press, 2009).

T. Babor et al., *Alcohol: No Ordinary Commodity* (2nd edition)
(Oxford: Oxford University Press, 2010).

Chapter 6: The future of addiction

D. Courtwright, *The Age of Addiction: How Bad Habits Became Big
Business* (Cambridge, MA: Harvard University Press, 2019).

K. Humphreys, V. Felbab-Brown, and J. Caulkins, "Opioids of the
masses: Stopping an American epidemic from going global,"
Foreign Affairs, 97, pp. 118–29 (2018).

The story of the Eloi and the Morlocks and their strange relationship
is a creation of H. G. Wells in his book *The Time Machine*
(London: William Heinemann, 1895).

Further reading

P. J. Cook, *Paying the Tab: The Costs and Benefits of Alcohol Control* (Princeton: Princeton University Press, 2017).

S. Darke, J. Lappin, and M. Farrell, *The Pocket Guide to Drugs and Health* (Sutton: Silverback Publishing, 2021).

G. E. Edwards, *Matters of Substance—Drugs, and why Everyone is a User* (New York: Thomas Dunne Books, 2005).

K. Humphreys and A. Lingford-Hughes, *Edwards' Treatment of Drinking Problems* (6th edition) (Cambridge: Cambridge University Press, 2016).

S. C. Miller, D. A. Fiellin, R. N. Rosenthal, and R. Saitz (eds), *Principles of Addiction Medicine* (6th edition) (Washington, DC: American Society of Addiction Medicine, 2019).

J. Orford, *Addiction Dilemmas: Family Experiences from Literature and Research and Their Lessons for Practice* (New York, Wiley & Sons, 2011).

A treasure trove of historical documents, interviews with leaders in the addiction field, and writings has been assembled by Bill White at <https://www.chestnut.org/william-white-papers/>.

Index

For the benefit of digital users, indexed terms that span two pages (e.g., 52–53) may, on occasion, appear on only one of those pages.

Addiction

EPIDEMIOLOGY
A Very Short Introduction
Rodolfo Saracci

Epidemiology has had an impact on many areas of medicine;
and lung cancer, to the origin and spread of new epidemics.
and lung cancer, to the origin and spread of new epidemics.
However, it is often poorly understood, largely due to
misrepresentations in the media. In this *Very Short Introduction*
Rodolfo Saracci dispels some of the myths surrounding the
study of epidemiology. He provides a general explanation of
the principles behind clinical trials, and explains the nature of
basic statistics concerning disease. He also looks at the ethical
and political issues related to obtaining and using information
concerning patients, and trials involving placebos.

AUTISM
A Very Short Introduction
Uta Frith

This *Very Short Introduction* offers a clear statement on what is currently known about autism and Asperger syndrome. Explaining the vast array of different conditions that hide behind these two labels, and looking at symptoms from the full spectrum of autistic disorders, it explores the possible causes for the apparent rise in autism and also evaluates the links with neuroscience, psychology, brain development, genetics, and environmental causes including MMR and Thimerosal. This short, authoritative, and accessible book also explores the psychology behind social impairment and savantism and sheds light on what it is like to live inside the mind of the sufferer.

HIV/AIDS
A Very Short Introduction
Alan Whiteside

HIV/AIDS is without doubt the worst epidemic to hit humankind since the Black Death. The first case was identified in 1981; by 2004 it was estimated that about 40 million people were living with the disease, and about 20 million had died. The news is not all bleak though. There have been unprecedented breakthroughs in understanding diseases and developing drugs. Because the disease is so closely linked to sexual activity and drug use, the need to understand and change behaviour has caused us to reassess what it means to be human and how we should operate in the globalising world. This *Very Short Introduction* provides an introduction to the disease, tackling the science, the international and local politics, the fascinating demographics, and the devastating consequences of the disease, and explores how we have — and must — respond.

'It won't make you an expert. But you'll know what you're talking about and you'll have a better idea of all the work we still have to do to wrestle this monster to the ground.'

Aids-free world website.

www.oup.com/vsi

SLEEP
A Very Short Introduction
Russell G. Foster & Steven W. Lockley

Why do we need sleep? What happens when we don't get enough? From the biology and psychology of sleep and the history of sleep in science, art, and literature; to the impact of a 24/7 society and the role of society in causing sleep disruption, this *Very Short Introduction* addresses the biological and psychological aspects of sleep, providing a basic understanding of what sleep is and how it is measured, looking at sleep through the human lifespan and the causes and consequences of major sleep disorders. Russell G. Foster and Steven W. Lockley go on to consider the impact of modern society, examining the relationship between sleep and work hours, and the impact of our modern lifestyle.

www.oup.com/vsi

FORENSIC PSYCHOLOGY
A Very Short Introduction
David Canter

Lie detection, offender profiling, jury selection, insanity in the law, predicting the risk of re-offending, the minds of serial killers and many other topics that fill news and fiction are all aspects of the rapidly developing area of scientific psychology broadly known as Forensic Psychology. *Forensic Psychology: A Very Short Introduction* discusses all the aspects of psychology that are relevant to the legal and criminal process as a whole. It includes explanations of criminal behaviour and criminality, including the role of mental disorder in crime, and discusses how forensic psychology contributes to helping investigate the crime and catching the perpetrators.

www.oup.com/vsi